Key Management Skills in Nursing

Edited by Roswyn A Brown and George Castledine

Deep vein thrombosis:
the silent killer

by
Ricky Autar

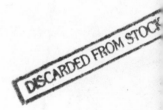

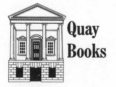

**Quay
Books**

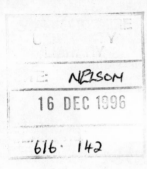
Quay Books, Division of Mark Allen Publishing Limited
Jesses Farm, Snow Hill, Dinton, Nr Salisbury, Wilts, SP3 5HN

©Mark Allen Publishing Ltd, 1996
ISBN 1-85642-110 4

British Library Cataloguing-in-Publication Data
A catalogue record for this book is available from the British
Library

Printed in the UK by Beshara Press, Cheltenham

Contents

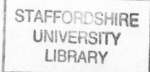

Deep vein thrombosis: the silent killer

Acknowledgements

Numerous people were instrumental in making this book a reality. Thanks go to Cathy, my wife and the children for their tolerance and forbearance. I am grateful to Alan Wood, subject specialist in Information Technology, for his advice in enabling me to produce a user friendly Autar DVT Scale.

Unreserved thanks are due to Roswyn Brown, Principal Lecturer at the University of Central England in Birmingham. She listened to me actively and patiently and her ongoing assistance and support enabled me to complete the manuscript.

The contributions of the nurses of varying levels of competence (novice to expert) who reviewed the chapters are acknowledged.

Finally, I am grateful to my nursing and teaching colleagues for their guidance with the contents and organisation of this book.

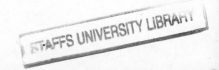

Foreword

This excellent book provides nurses with an effective tool for establishing the level of risk of deep vein thrombosis to which particular client groups are exposed. As Ricky Autar rightly points out the current array of assessment strategies that are available are laboratory-bases, expensive to use, require physically invasive procedures to provide appropriate haematological specimens and, finally, are the exclusive prerogative of the medical staff.

The publication of the Autar DVT Scale is timely in that it will enable nurses (and indeed other members of the health care team, such as physiotherapists) to make a major contribution to the prevention of this distressing, costly and potentially fatal condition. The Scale is inexpensive to use in terms of staff time and documentation material. It is easy to utilise and understand. It could make a major contribution to the further harmonisation between the work roles of nurses and doctors and enhance the notion of collaborative care. It epitomises the part that nurses can play in health promotion and disease prevention. In addition, the story that this development tells is about the advancement of nursing practice. Ricky Autar has demonstrated very ably how he has combined the sub-roles of education, research and innovation in the 'pursuit of advanced practice'. This has been in the spirit of pushing back the boundaries and demonstrating the impact of creative professional nursing practice which is not only efficient and effective but caring too.

R A Brown
Director of Studies, MSc in Advanced Nursing Practice, University of Central England in Birmingham

Preface

Ask nurses about the complications of bedrest and they will say that deep vein thrombosis (DVT) is one of them. It is now considered negligent not to provide thromboprophylaxis for clients at risk (Parker-Williams and Vickers, 1991). Both the National Institute of Health (NIH, 1986) and the European Consensus Statement (1991) recommend the need for vigorous prophylaxis based on the three risk categories: Low, Moderate and High. There is no single, universal efficacious prophylaxis. Low dose Heparin (LDH) may be appropriate to some clients 'at risk' and risky and contraindicated in others. For prophylaxis to be efficacious, it must be tailored to the clients in the light of risk category assessment.

Current assessment methods documenting clients at potential risk of DVT only provides a very crude index of risk measurement. A gap exists in this area of assessment. The fatality associated with DVT has created an urgent need to develop a simple, easy-to-use method which identifies these individuals before a DVT crisis occurs. The Autar DVT Scale has been developed as a risk calculator to enable nurses of all levels of competence — novice to expert — to address this problem. This book is the outcome of a research project submitted to the University of Central England in Birmingham (UCE) as a requirement for the MSc in Advanced Nursing Practice Course.

Deep vein thrombosis: the silent killer

Chapter 1

Introduction

This thing called deep vein thrombosis (DVT): double trouble

It is many years ago now but I still recall this experience with some apprehension. At the time I was undertaking clinical experience on a surgical ward as a junior student nurse. Mr Harry Payne, aged 45 years, was making a good recovery following a cholecystectomy. His impending discharge plan was being finalised when it was noted that he was limping due to a painful and swollen left calf. This was duly reported to the house officer who suspected deep vein thrombosis. To confirm the provisional diagnosis a venogram was requested. While on bedrest waiting for the venography, Mr Payne had a sudden excruciating chest pain and collapsed. I watched helplessly as the resuscitation team went into action. Double trouble: the DVT had propagated into a fatal pulmonary embolism. All attempts to revive Mr Payne failed.

The impact of the cost in terms of pain, human misery and sheer economics struck me forcibly and, as a novice, I felt powerless. DVT is usually preventable and as an advanced practitioner, I realised that in collaboration with colleagues, I could push back the boundaries and do something about this unexpected killer: hence, the Autar DVT Risk Assessment Scale.

Deep vein thrombosis: what is it?

Deep vein thrombosis (DVT), as the term implies, is the formation of a clot in the deep vein. The deep veins are so-called because they are embedded intramuscularly in the deep fascia in contrast to the superficial veins which are extramuscular, outside the deep fascia (Figure 1.1). The deep and superficial veins are connected by communicating veins, also know as 'perforators'. Deep veins tend to thrombose while superficial veins are prone to varicose. The varicose veins become dilated and tortuous due to the damage to the vein valves caused by high back pressure.

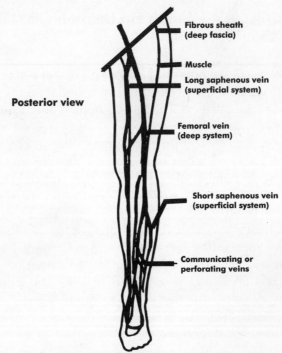

Figure 1-1 : Deep, superficial and communicating leg veins

While deep veins are present throughout the body, venous thrombosis commonly occurs in the deep veins of the legs.

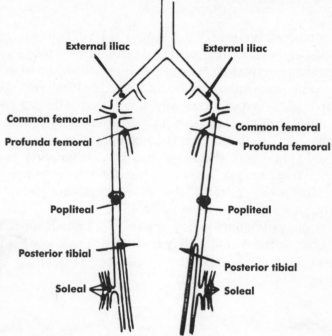

Figure 1-2: Primary sites of DVT in deep leg veins

Six primary sites are recognised and these are illustrated in Figure 1.2.

Deep vein thrombosis: the scope of the problem

Nightingale (1869) famously advised that hospitals should do patients no harm. It is, therefore, with some irony that DVT has been described as a 'disease of hospitalised patients' (Douglas, 1978). It is a condition which can have serious and sometimes fatal consequences. Complications of DVT are listed below:

- Pulmonary embolism
- Postphlebitis syndrome
- Recurrence of DVT

Pulmonary embolism (PE), a sequel of DVT, is a potentially lethal complication. It is a serious cause of mortality in both surgical and non-surgical patients and is still detected in 10% of hospital autopsies (Sandler and Martin, 1989). PE occurs when a detached clot, usually associated with leg veins, migrates through the heart to the pulmonary circulation (Figure 1.3). This serious vascular complication compromises the individual gas exchange and the obstruction causes infarction in the area. The size of the clot and artery occluded determine what occurs. If the clot is large enough to block the pulmonary arteries, sudden death occurs. If the clot blocks one pulmonary artery or a smaller branch, death may not occur or the embolus may cause death in a few hours to several days as the clot grows with the pulmonary blood vessels.

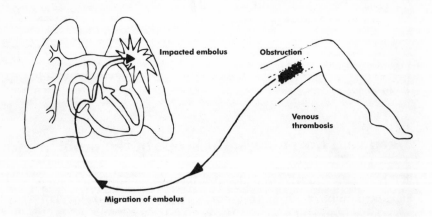

Figure 1-3: Pulmonary embolism as a sequel of DVT

A patient with a previous history of DVT is not only highly likely to experience a recurrence (Kakkar *et al*, 1970) but may go on to develop further complications, such as postphlebitis syndrome (Dalen *et al*, 1986). This is a state of venous insufficiency and causes recanalisation of the major blood clots, which eventually destroys the valve. In recanalisation, blood flowing through a previously blocked vein is restored. This is brought about by the action of white blood cells (phagocytes) which digest the thrombus to establish new endothelium lined channels. This process or recanalisation is illustrated in Figure 1.4.

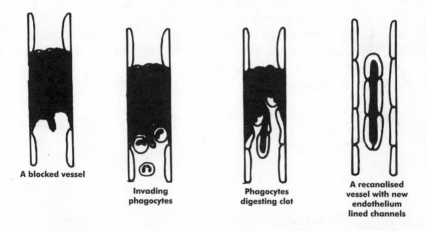

Figure 1-4: Process of recanalisation (adapted from Lakhani *et al*, 1993)

A recanalised vessel is never as good as new. In the long-term, as a consequence of recanalisation and valve destruction, the muscular venous pump fails. This leads to pooling of blood and high venous pressure in the calf. Venous stasis from the pooling blood is a major factor in deep vein thrombus formation, while the high pressure predisposes to varicosity of the superficial veins. A reported DVT incidence of 48% is associated with varicose veins (Schaub *et al*, 1975).

How reliable is a DVT clinical (medical) diagnosis?

A clinical diagnosis of DVT is notoriously unreliable even to the most watchful observer. Barnes (1982) found approximately 50% inaccuracy when using the Homan's sign to make a clinical diagnosis of DVT. In Homan's sign, pain is elicited on forceful dorsiflexion (bending the foot and toes upwards). DVT is not often suspected until it has propagated or caused PE. In a five-year retrospective study, Sandler and Martin (1989) recorded 195 deaths from PE in a general hospital. At post-mortem, DVT was confirmed in 162 patients but 157 patients were not diagnosed before death: a hidden and silent killer in 81% of cases.

Table 1.1 illustrates the reliability of clinical diagnosis:

Table 1.1: The reliability of clinical diagnosis

Diagnostic findings	No of patients	%
Death by PE	195	100
DVT found at autopsy	162	83
DVT not found at autopsy	12	6
DVT not known at autopsy	21	11
DVT not diagnosed before death	157	81
DVT not suspected before death	38	19

Source of data: Sandler and Martin, 1989

The nurse's role in primary prevention

With a remarkably high incidence of DVT being described as 'silent' — asymptomatic and unsuspected — morbidity and mortality can be reduced only by primary prevention. This can be achieved by a systematic, comprehensive and objective risk assessment strategy, followed by appropriate interventions (The Kendall Company, 1992). It is now considered an act of negligence not to provide venous thromboprophylaxis for patients at risk of DVT (Parker-Williams and Vickers, 1991).

Since previous DVT increases the likelihood of recurrence by 68% (Kakkar *et al*, 1970), the essence of DVT management is in its prevention. In exercising their professional accountability, all registered nurses must:

'...ensure that no action or omission on your part, or within your sphere of responsibility, is detrimental to the interests, condition or safety of patients and clients' (UKCC, 1992).

Nurses are key people not only in delivering and co-ordinating care but also in facilitating health education strategies. Therefore, they are well placed to assess and implement preventative measures. The risk of DVT is greater after an acute or exacerbated illness, trauma and surgery where health deficits are at their greatest and patients become highly dependent on nursing support. Although definitive treatment is the province of physicians, nurses have a clear role in the primary prevention of DVT. After all, in practice it is the nursing team who administer any prescribed prophylactic and therapeutic protocol on a day-to-day basis.

DVT risk assessment

A review of the medical literature has highlighted a number of predicting instruments formulated to identify clients at risk (Clayton *et al*, 1976; Crandon *et al*, 1980; Lowe *et al*, 1982; Sue-Ling *et al*, 1986, Caprini *et al*, 1991). All of the above prognostic indexes are calculated from some equation combining clinical factors and blood tests. Laboratory tests to determine blood viscosity, euglobulin lysis time and estimation of antithrombin 111 concentration are some of the battery of serological investigations for hypercoagulability. This dependence on laboratory testing to enable a comprehensive assessment and diagnosis is probably the reason why the medical indexes have not been widely and successfully implemented. Laboratory tests can be initiated only by medical staff and therefore exclude a significant element of the health care team, such as nurses, from contributing to risk reduction. This monopoly of risk assessment tools has previously created an embargo on the contribution of the nursing workforce to the assessment of risk and therefore to the reduction of actual DVT episodes. An effective and easily applied assessment tool is often a simple instrument. This view is supported by Ruckley (1985) who claims that simple criteria and accessible data based on clinical risk factors, such as age or the type of surgery, are more likely to be adopted by clinicians as well as other health care members, including nurses, physiotherapists and occupational therapists.

Nursing assessment is a domain of practice which is undergoing considerable change and refinement. A variety of nursing instruments are now available in the clinical area, enabling nurses to carry out systematic, comprehensive, nursing diagnoses. Norton *et al*, (1962) introduced the pressure sore risk scale and this risk calculator was later developed by Gosnell (1973) and Waterlow (1985). The Glasgow Coma Scale (Teasdale, 1975) to assess the level of consciousness, the Barthel Index (Mahoney and Barthel,

1965) to assess the activities of daily living and a number of pain-o-meters or pain scales are analogues of the wide range of instruments which are available for use in the clinical area. An investigation into risk assessment of clients for risk of DVT confirms inconsistency in the assessment of practice and this is often based on subjective judgement or pre-printed core care plans (Autar, 1994). A blanket nursing diagnosis of potential problems of DVT provides only a very crude index of measurement of the problem. It fails to address the nature of risk in an individual in the context of multifactorial aetiology. Unless risk is identified by degree or category and tailored to the individual, preventative measures are likely to be inappropriate and therefore ineffective.

Identifying those at risk as well as those who are not is of equal importance. It allows the targeting of limited resources and ensures that nursing action is individualised and founded on rationale and not ritual. A risk assessment system based on clearly defined criteria and readily available information from clinical nursing history can yield an index of low, moderate and high risk of DVT. Because high risk patients are easily recognised, low to moderate risk candidates are often missed. Low risk patients carry less than 10% risk of DVT, rising to 40% for moderate risk categories. As high as 80% DVT incidence has been reported for the high risk group (European Consensus Statement, 1991; Grace, 1993).

The cost of utilising preventative practices based on risk assessment is considerably less than the cost of treating the problem once it occurs (The Kendall Company, 1992). With increasing pressure to reduce cost and hospital stays, the National Institutes of Health (1986) and the European Consensus Statement (1991) strongly recommend the implementation of a prophylactic protocol based on risk assessment and risk categories. The recommended methods for those assessed at different levels of risk are listed in Table 1.2 (see page 10).

The array of assessment strategies available to identify patients at risk of DVT continues to be laboratory-dependent, expensive, requires invasive procedures and remains the exclusive prerogative of the medical staff. The purpose of this book is to discuss the development and application of the first nursing DVT risk calculation — the Autar DVT Scale. This development has been directed at enabling nurses and other members of the health care team, such as physiotherapists and medical staff, to harmonise and enhance the concept of collaborative care.

Table 1.2: Anti-thrombotic prophylaxis strategy

Risk category	Recommended prophylaxis
High risk: >40%	
Major orthopaedic surgery	Graduated compression stockings
Fractured pelvis, hip, leg	Adjusted dose Heparin
Major surgery in patients with malignancy	Intermittent pneumatic compression
Major surgery in patients with history of venous thromboembolism or >60 years-old	
Lower limb paralysis	
Moderate risk: 5–40%	
Major surgery in patients >40 years-old not in high risk category	Graduated compression stockings
Major surgery or lower limb surgery in patients on contraceptive pill	Low dose Heparin

Risk category	Recommended prophylaxis
Major medical illness with prolonged immobilisation (malignancy, cardica, inflammatory bowel disease)	
Low risk: <5%	
Minor surgery (<30 minutes) with no risk factor	Graduated compression stockings
Major surgery in patients <40 years-old with no risk factors	

Summary

- Deep vein thrombosis poses a threat to recovery and can seriously damage the health of hospitalised clients
- Pulmonary embolism, a potentially lethal complication of DVT, is still detected in 10% of hospital autopsies
- DVT is preventable and the cost of treating clients with the problem is considerably more than preventative practices
- Although treatment of DVT is the province of the physicians, nurses have a clear role in its primary prevention
- The practice of applying a blanket diagnosis to potential DVT provides only a very crude index of risk measurement. On the other hand, a nursing assessment strategy tailored to the individual and based on the cumulative effects of risk factors in DVT can yield a prognostic index of low, moderate or high risk category
- Assessment of clients by risk category enables the application of a prophylactic regime commensurate with the nature and degree of risk

● It is now considered negligent not to provide thrombophylaxis for clients at risk. Both the National Institutes of Health and the European Consensus Statement recommend DVT prophylaxis derived from risk assessment and risk categorisation.

References

Autar R (1994) *Nursing assessment of clients at risk of deep vein thrombosis (DVT). The Autar DVT Scale.* Unpublished MSc Dissertation. University of Central England, Birmingham

Barnes RW (1982) Current status of non-invasive tests in the diagnosis of venous disease. *Surg Clin N Am* **62(3)**: 484–500

Caprini JA, Arcelus JI, Hasty JH, Tamhane AC, Fabrega F (1991) Clinical assessment of venous thromboembolic risk in surgical patients. *Seminar in Thrombosis and Hemostasis* **17(3)**: 304–11

Clayton JK, Anderson JA, McNicol GP (1976) Preoperative prediction of post-operative deep vein thrombosis. *Br Med J* **2**: 910–2

Crandon AJ, Peel KR, Anderson JA, Thompson V, McNicol GP (1980) Post-operative deep vein thrombosis: identifying high risk patients. *Br Med J* **7**: 343–4

Dalen JE, Paraskos J, Ochene IS, Alpert JS, Hirsh J (1986) Venous thromboembolism: scope of the problem. *Chest* **89(5)**: 370s–3s

Douglas A (1978) Venous thrombosis and pulmonary embolism: a disease of the hospitals. *Nurs Times* **147(17)**: 44–6

European Consensus Statement (1991) *Prevention of Venous Thromboembolism*. Med-Orion Publishing, London

Grace R (1993) Thromboprophylaxis: a review. *Br J Hos Med* **49(10)**: 720–6

Gosnell DJ (1973) An assessment tool to identify pressure sores. *Nurs Res* **22**: 55–9

Kakkar VV, Howe C, Nicolaides AN, Renney JTG, Clark MB (1970) Deep vein thrombosis of the legs. Is there a high risk group? *Am J Surg* **120**: 527–30

Kendall Company (1992) *The Guide to Protocol Development for the Prevention of Deep Vein Thrombosis and Pulmonary Embolism*. Kendall Healthcare Products, Europe

Lakhani SK, Dilly SA (1993) *Basic pathology: an introduction to the mechanism of disease*. Edward Arnold, London

Lowe GD, McArdle BM, Carter DC *et al* (1982) Prediction and selective prophylaxis of venous thrombosis in elective gastro-intestinal surgery. *Lancet* **1**: 409–12

Mahoney I, Barthel DW (1965) Functional Evaluation in the Barthel Index. *Maryland State Med J* **14**: 61–5

National Institutes of Health (1986) Consensus development conference on the prevention of venous thrombosis and pulmonary embolism. *J Am Med Ass* **25b**: 744–9

Nightingale F (1869) *Notes on Nursing : What is it and it is not?* Republished 1980. Churchill Livingstone, Edinburgh

Norton D, McClaren R, Exton-Smith AN (1962) *An Investigation of Geriatric Nursing Problems in Hospital*. National Corporation for the Care of Old People, London

Parker-Williams J, Vickers (1991) Major orthopaedic surgery on the leg and thromboembolism. *Br Med J* **303**: 531–2

Ruckley C (1985) Protection against thromboembolism. *Br J Surg* **72(6)**: 421–2

Sandler DA, Martin JF (1989) Autopsy proven pulmonary embolism in hospital patients: are we detecting enough deep vein thrombosis? *J Roy Soc Med* **82**: 203–5

Schaub N, Duckert F, Fridrick R, Gruber UF (1975) Post-operative venous thrombosis. *Lagenbeck Arch Chir* **340**: 23

Sue-Ling HM, Johnson D, McMahon MJ, Philips PR (1986) Preoperative identification of patients at risk of deep vein thrombosis after elective major abdominal surgery. *Lancet* **1**: 1173–6

Teasdale GM (1975) Assessing conscious level. *Nurs Times* **71(24)**: 914–7

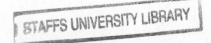

UKCC (1992) *The Code of Professional Conduct*. UKCC, London

Waterlow J (1985) A risk assessment card. *Nurs Times* **81(49)**: 51–5

Chapter 2

Theoretical framework

A better understanding of the aetiology and pathogenesis of DVT helps in the early identification of those at risk. This can reduce morbidity and mortality by implementing appropriate preventative measures (Nicolaides and Irving, 1975).

Protective mechanisms in the normal vascular systems

A number of mechanisms exist which protect individuals from DVT. A review of these mechanisms suggests explanations as to why some patients are more susceptible to DVT.

Clot prevention

In normal vascular systems various clot prevention mechanisms operate as follows:

- The *endothelium* is a simple squamous epithelium which lines the lumen of all blood vessels. The smoothness of the endothelium prevents contact activation of the intrinsic clotting system. This is due to the inner surface of the endothelium being coated with a layer of glycocalyx

- *Glycocalyx* is a mucopolysaccharide which repels clotting factors and platelets. Therefore any damage to the endothelium will tip the balance towards thrombosis

- *Thrombomodulin* is another clot prevention mechanism. It is a protein which binds with thrombin to slow down the clotting process. It also activates plasma protein C which has an anticoagulant action

- *Heparin* is a naturally occurring anticoagulant but its concentration in blood is too slight to have any significant effect

- *Fibrin threads* formed during the clotting process and antithrombin III, an alpha globulin, are two powerful neutralisers of thrombin

- *Alpha macroglobulin*, a binding agent, inhibits the proteolytic action of several clotting factors until the latter are destroyed.

Table 2.1: Normal clot prevention mechanism

Mechanism	Effect
Endothelium	Prevents contact activation of the clotting system
Glycocalyx	Repels clotting factors and platelets
Thrombomodulin	Binds with Thrombin to slow the clotting process
Heparin	Anticoagulates
Fibrin threads	Neutralise Thrombin
Antithrombin III	Neutralises Thrombin
Alpha macroglobulin	Inhibits proteolytic action of several clotting factors

Fibrinolysis

Fibrinolysis is a system which is concerned with the dissolution of clots as well as the prevention of thrombi formation (Poller, 1993). Plasma proteins contain an euglobulin called plasminogen. When a clot is formed, plasminogen is trapped in it. The trapped plasminogen remains inactive until the injured tissue releases tissue plasminogen activator which converts plasminogen into plasmin. Plasmin is a powerful enzyme which digests fibrin threads and destroys some clotting factors.

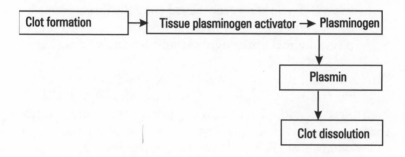

Figure 2-1: Process of fibrinolysis

Pathogenesis of deep vein thrombosis

Virchow's triad

Fitting tribute is due to Rudolph Virchow (1821–1902) for his pioneering work in providing a sound understanding of the pathophysiology of DVT. The triad of factors that are associated with DVT, as first explained by Virchow, are:

1. *Changes in the vessel wall due to intimal damage of the endothelium lining the vessel.* Injury to the endothelium may be caused by trauma, fracture, thermal injury, surgical procedures and

instrumentation and inflammatory process by endotoxin. Microtears in the endothelium can also be caused by venous stasis and overdistension.

2. *Change in blood flow due to venous stasis.* Immobility is one of the major contributors to venous stasis. Venous stasis causes abnormal blood flow in valve pockets which are potential sites for clot formation.

3. *Changes in the composition of blood due to hypercoagulability.* Increased coagulation is caused by increased platelet activity and/or a decrease in physiological anticoagulant and fibrinolytic activity.

Virchow's seminal work makes it possible and practical to examine the multifactorial context for identifying those at high risk and so allows for appropriate venous thromboprophylaxis to be applied. The triad of risk factors in the genesis of DVT is illustrated in Figure 2.2.

Stasis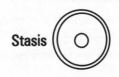

Coagulation factors 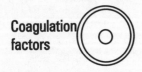 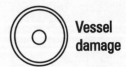 Vessel damage

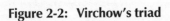

Figure 2-2: Virchow's triad

Risk factors in DVT

A number of clinical circumstances increase the risk of deep vein thrombosis. There is substantial evidence (Kakkar *et al*, 1970) which demonstrates that a number of clinical factors increase the susceptibility to DVT. The well-documented high risk factors are listed below:

- Surgery
- Trauma
- Increasing age
- Obesity
- Immobility
- Specific DVT risk factors
- High risk diseases

Each of the above risk factors will now be examined in the context of their uniqueness and potential weighting for causing DVT. Included in this examination will be the contribution that an understanding of the risk factors will make to the development of the Autar DVT Risk Scale. A rationale will be provided for the inclusion or omission of particular risk factors from the Autar Scale.

Surgery

Nature of surgery

The nature of surgery determines different weighting risks. Major surgery is defined as a procedure on a patient requiring more than 30 minutes of general anaesthesia (Goucke, 1989; Moser, 1989) and carries higher risk. Flanc *et al* (1969) reported a DVT incidence of 44% for major surgery in comparison to only 15% for minor surgery lasting less than 30 minutes. Kakkar *et al* (1970) studied 203 patients and detected 33.1% DVT for major surgery and 25% for minor surgery. Incidence of DVT is between 0.2–2.0% for elective surgery, rising to 2.7% for emergency operation.

Duration of surgery

There is also a linear relationship between DVT and the duration of surgery. Incidence of DVT in surgery of less than 2 hours is 20% and 46.7% for 2–3 hours, escalating to 62.5% in procedure over 3 hours. Table 2.2 (Borrow and Goldson, 1981) outlines the association between duration of surgery and the incidence of DVT(%).

Table 2.2: Association between duration of surgery and incidence of DVT(%)

Duration of surgery	Incidence (%)
< 2 hours	20.0
2–3 hours	46.7
> 3 hours	62.5

Source of data: Borrow and Goldson, 1981

Types of surgery

Some surgical procedures are associated with comparatively higher incidence of DVT than others. The risk following orthopaedic surgery is greater than other procedures, partly because of the trauma to the tissue surrounding the deep vein and partly due to the difficulty in moving the injured limb to maintain venous return. One in two patients may develop DVT after total hip replacement (Parker-Williams and Vickers, 1991). Manipulation of the leg during total hip replacement causes distortion and occlusion of the femoral vein and is claimed to cause DVT (Stamatakis *et al*, 1977). Table 2.3 illustrates the incidence of deep vein thrombosis associated with the different types of surgery.

Table 2.3: Incidence of deep vein thrombosis associated with surgery

Types	Incidence of DVT (%)
Orthopaedic	
Knee replacement	84
Hip replacement	30–65
Open menisectomy	20–25
General surgery	
Abdominal	3–51
Thoracic	26
Gynaecological	7–45
Retropubic prostatectomy	24–51
Transvesical prostatectomy	7–10
Neurosurgical	29–43

Sources of data: Madden and Hume, 1976; European Consensus Statement, 1991; Grace, 1993

Surgery as a high risk factor

Venous stasis, increased coagulability and vessel trauma are all present perioperatively. Virchow's triad of factors are also present in surgery, making it the primary risk factor in DVT.

Venous stasis: Stasis is caused by pre- and post-operative immobilisation and general anaesthesia with concurrent loss of venous pump function. Thiopentone induction anaesthesia also produces venous stasis.

Increased coagulability: During surgery the enzyme thromboplastin is released, increasing the coagulability of blood. Surgical intervention also brings about changes in the fibrinolytic system. Delayed fibrolysis following surgery can have a catastrophic effect by causing pulmonary embolism.

Vessel trauma: Trauma to the vessel wall and increased thrombocytosis (raised platelet count) favour the formation of thrombi.

Trauma as a risk factor

The reported incidence of DVT in patients with trauma varies between 20% and 90% (Shackford and Moser, 1988). This high incidence is possibly the result of skewed data due to the inclusion of patients with hip fracture. Patients with a fractured neck of femur often belong to a group of patients who are elderly with coexisting medical problems associated with thrombogenesis.

Coon (1976) claims that all patients with accident trauma, irrespective of sites, carry some risk of DVT. Head or chest injuries carry 25% risk and spinal injuries 14%. Pelvic injuries are reported at 22% with the incidence for tibial and femoral fractures rising to the highest in the trauma nomenclature. They range between 40% and 60% (Coon, 1976). In hip fracture, DVT risk starts at the time of injury due to the nature and site of the trauma. In hip surgery, DVT can be caused by accidental damage to the endothelium caused by manipulation during the procedure. This is thought to be partly responsible for deep femoral thrombosis (Stamatakis *et al*, 1977).

The highest incidence of DVT reported in injury to the lower limb is due to venous stasis, intimal vessel wall damage and hypercoagulability, which are the triad predisposing to DVT (Wheeler, 1988). In lower limb trauma, due to either application of plaster of Paris or external fixators, complex wound or traction, the commonly applied DVT prophylaxis, such as graded compression stockings and intermittent pneumatic compression, cannot be implemented. With such complex wounds caused by compound fracture, anticoagulation is not always advised as it may interfere with the healing process or increase the risk of haemorrhage. Enforced immobility due to lower limb trauma is also a contributory factor in the pathogenesis of deep vein thrombosis.

An extensive literature review by Shackford and Moser (1988) on trauma clients yielded eight studies firmly establishing some variability in the incidence of DVT. The analysis of the eight studies is reported in Table 2.4.

Table 2.4: Incidence of DVT in trauma patients

Study	Year	No of Patients	%
Sevitt and Gallagher	1961	125	81
Freeark et al	1967	124	44
Nylander and Semb	1972	15	7
Silver et al	1980	100	18
Brach et al	1977	10	9
Rossi et al	1980	18	13
Willen et al	1982	38	8
Myllynen et al	1985	37	18

Some groups of young trauma patients are also at high risk due to the types of injuries sustained. Incidence of 18–90% is reported for patients with spinal injuries as documented in Table 2.5.

Table 2.5: DVT incidence after spinal injury

Study	No of Patients	No of DVT	%
Servitt and Gallaher	2	1	50
Silver et al	100	18	18
Brach et al	10	9	90
Rossi et al	18	13	72
Myllynen et al	23	18	78

The low DVT incidence of 18% reported in the Silver *et al* study (1980) may be due to the implementation of prophylactic anticoagulation in 68% of the subjects.

Increasing age

Post-mortem and clinical studies have demonstrated that the incidence of DVT rises with advancing age. Age is the most important intrinsic factor and the risk rises after the age of forty (Nicolaides and Irving, 1975). The increased frequency with advancing age may be partly due to the increased likelihood of coexisting medical illnesses or surgery and may also be associated with reduced mobility. As age increases, the soleal veins increase in number, size and tortuosity. The calf muscle mass decreases, thus both changes reduce the efficiency of the venous pump and contribute to a decrease in the rate of venous return from the lower limbs.

DVT is reduced considerably in children, with a clinical prevalence of 1–2 per 10000 admissions to a children's hospital (Coon, 1976). Even when DVT occurs, it is usually associated with conditions, such as trauma, leg or foot surgery, sepsis or femoral vein cannulation (Jones and MacIntyre, 1975). No venous thrombosis or embolism was reported under the age of fourteen (OPCS, 1990). The relationship between increasing age and the occurrence of

DVT is not clearly understood. Phlebosclerosis or narrowing and loss of elasticity of the veins due to old age has been described. The linear relationship between increasing age and DVT is listed under the International Classification of Disease (ICD) number 453 and illustrated in Table 2.6.

Table 2.6: Increasing age and associated venous embolism and thrombosis: International Classification of Disease (ICD) 453, 1990

Age groups	Total recorded cases
45–49	11
50–54	12
55–59	19
60–64	54
65–69	100
70–74	123
75–79	205

Source of data: OPCS (1990) Cause of mortality statistic

Several medical predictive indexes have been constructed to predict clients at risk of DVT (Clayton *et al*, 1976; Crandon *et al*, 1980; Lowe *et al*, 1982; Sue-Ling *et al*, 1986; Caprini *et al*, 1991). Of the variables included in their prognostic indexes, age was a significant and powerful predictor of DVT.

Obesity

Obese patients are at greater risk of developing DVT than their lean counterparts. Among women matched for age and parity, it was found that women who developed DVT were about 10 lbs (4.5 kg) heavier than those who did not (Vessey and Doll, 1969).

Obesity predisposes to DVT: a pendulous abdomen, in particular, mechanically increases intra-abdominal pressure and interferes with venous return. A decrease in the fibrinolytic activity is also reported in obese patients (Poller, 1993). Table 2.7 illustrates the incidence of DVT in different weight groups.

Table 2.7: Association between weight and incidence of DVT

Weight	DVT	No DVT	Total
Overweight	23	25	48
Average	21	56	77
Underweight	17	61	78

Source of data: Kakkar et al, 1970

It may be argued that obesity commonly leads to relative immobility in the post-operative period. In the Kakkar *et al* study (1970), obese patients appear to have twice the normal risk of developing DVT post-operatively. Obesity as a high risk factor for DVT was further substantiated by Schaub *et al* (1975). Of the 95 subjects studied, DVT was detected in 52 obese patients as diagnosed by routine 125/Fibrinogen scanning.

Immobility

Venous return to the heart requires the combined efforts of cardiac contraction, respiratory inspiration and expiration. The calf muscle pump is the powerhouse forcing venous blood towards the heart. Lack of movement of the calf muscle causes a drop in venous return.

Immobility causes stasis and is a major contributor of DVT. When normal venous pump function is lost as a result of confinement to bed, venous stasis manifests itself in at least two forms. First of all, there is an actual decrease in the linear velocity of blood, affecting venous return from the lower extremities. Secondly, this is followed by dilation of the vein delaying further venous return (Caprini *et al*, 1988).

Sharnoff and Rosenberg (1964) compared immobilised patients who have undergone open reduction and internal fixation (ORIF) with mobile patients who have undergone prostatectomies. The conclusion drawn from this experimental study is that immobility is a potent and a discriminatory factor in the development of DVT. Immobility as a high risk factor was supported by the Miller *et al* study (1976) in which there was a marked reduction in the incidence of DVT in patients with myocardial infarction who were mobilised within 2–3 days of the onset of their attack. As a matter of course, coronary care units now favour the regime of early mobilisation of clients following myocardial infarction. There is also a striking relationship between the length of confinement to bed and the occurrence of DVT. It rises from zero after two days in bed to 100% after fourteen days (Sevitt and Gallagher, 1969).

In a study of 109 non-surgical bedridden patients, Kierkegaard *et al* (1987) reported a total incidence of DVT of 13%. The study of immobility was restricted to the first eight days following admission. Apparently, DVT occurred throughout the period of the study and this finding contradicts previous studies which claim that DVT normally occurs in the first few days after operation following immobility. This might explain why only 13% of DVT were reported. Kierkegaard *et al* (1987) claim that a much higher incidence of DVT would have been reported if the patients had been studied for a longer period.

In a comparative study between medical patients and those who have undergone surgery, compelling evidence indicates that bedrest and immobility is a causative factor, whereas surgery *per se* is indirectly responsible (Murray *et al*, 1970).

The Lassen and Borris (1991) case control study to evaluate the influence of immobility on patients after hip surgery, confirms the importance of early mobilisation in DVT thromboprophylaxis. Incidence of DVT in patients with hip surgery is usually between 48–74% (Madden and Hume, 1976). The patients in the experimental group who were mobilised on the fourth day had an incidence of 23% DVT compared with 75% in the control group whose mobilisation was delayed to the ninth day. In brief, there is conclusive evidence that immobility is a high risk factor in the causation of DVT.

Specific DVT risk factors

Oral contraceptives

Contraceptive methods are judged by their effectiveness, acceptability and freedom from side-effects. Oral contraceptives remain the most popular method of fertility control but are not without side-effects.

Controlled investigations (Sartwell *et al*, 1969; Vessey and Doll, 1970) are overwhelmingly supportive of the evidence that oestrogens increase the risk of DVT. Oral contraceptive therapy causes hypercoagulability of blood by increasing the level of fibrinogen, clotting factors VII, VIII, IX and X as well as a decrease in antithrombin activity. Oral contraceptives also cause venous stasis by their vasodilation action. Investigation of the relation between oral contraceptives and DVT (Vessey and Doll, 1970) confirms that 1 in every 2000 women using oral contraceptives developed DVT compared with 1 in every 20 000 not using them. Vessey and Doll (1970) also reported DVT occurrence as being 2.5 times greater in women aged 35–44 years than those aged 20–34 years.

Currently a progressive reduction in the dose of oestrogen to less than 50 micrograms, backed by better supervision have reduced risk of DVT still further. Porter *et al* (1985) in a follow-up of 65000 women in Seattle, suggest a relative risk of 2.8. Risk of DVT in women taking oral contraceptives during the month prior to surgery or trauma, appears to increase 4–6 fold (Sartwell and Stolley, 1982). To minimise the risk, it is recommended that women scheduled for surgery, should stop taking oral contraceptives 3–4 weeks prior to hospitalisation (BNF, 1994). When discontinuation of oral contraception is not possible and the clients admitted are still on oestrogen-containing pills, prophylactic subcutaneous heparin is recommended.

Pregnancy and puerperium

Normal pregnancy brings about homeostatic changes. An increase in coagulation factors, such as raised fibrinogen, platelets and suppressed fibrolysis, serve to combat the danger of haemorrhage at delivery. Equally, pregnancy raises the risk of developing DVT. Like obesity, a pendulous abdomen in pregnancy increases intra-abdominal pressure and interferes with venous return. The relative risk of DVT and pulmonary embolism in women who are pregnant and postpartum is 5.5 times greater than in non-pregnant and non-puerperal women not taking oral contraceptives (Coon, 1976).

In the triennium 1976–1978, 47 deaths were coded to pulmonary embolism following DVT, with one third occurring in the antenatal period (DHSS, 1982). In the triennium 1988–1990, 33 maternal deaths from pulmonary embolism were coded to thrombosis; of the reported maternal deaths 24 were from pulmonary embolism — 13 antepartum and 11 postpartum. In the 11 deaths, four of the women were aged 35 years or over and four weighed over 96 kg. The Enquiring Task Force on Maternal Deaths (DoH 1994) concluded that gross overweight and increasing   age augment the risk of thromboembolism.

The puerperium is the period immediately following delivery until the reproductive organs return to their non-pregnant state. It usually lasts 6–8 weeks. Within this time is the lying-in period, defined by the Central Midwives Board as a period of not less than 10 days and not more than

28 days after the birth of the baby. Although the oestrogen levels are considerably reduced during puerperium, they remain higher than normal. The plasma fluid composition is also reduced and coagulability is therefore enhanced.

High risk diseases

Ulcerative colitis

Ulcerative colitis is a chronic inflammatory bowel disease (IBD) in which part or the whole of the large bowel becomes diffusely inflamed with a haemorrhagic tendency.

The association between DVT and chronic ulcerative colitis was first documented by Edwards and Truelove (1964). Overall, a low incidence of 1.3–6.4 has been reported in inflammatory bowel disease. Physiological changes, such as an increase in clotting factor VIII and fibrinogen concentration occur in response to the haemorrhagic tendency. Chronic inflammatory bowel diseases are associated with hypercoagulability and elevation of clotting factors and platelets, favouring the formation of thrombi (Wyshock *et al*, 1988).

Haematological conditions

DVT is often a complication of polycythaemia, sickle cell anaemia and haemolytic anaemia. All of the above haematological conditions are characterised by increase in blood viscosity, persistent elevation of platelet count and venous stasis, creating an internal environment which favours the formation of thrombi.

Cardiac conditions

Clinical and pathological studies report a relationship between cardiovascular diseases and venous thromboembolism. The frequency of DVT and pulmonary embolism is 3.5 times greater in patients with cardiovascular disease than in patients who do not suffer from heart disease (Coon, 1976). Patients with atrial fibrillation and congestive heart failure are particularly at risk and an incidence of 10–20% has been recorded. In patients with acute myocardial infarction, 37% of incidences of DVT has been detected (Maurer *et al*, 1971). Heart disease is associated with cardiac arrhythmias and reduced mobility which influence venous return and cardiac output. The relationship between cardiac conditions and the incidence of DVT has also been linked to other common risk factors, such as immobility, obesity and smoking. Simmons *et al* (1973) studied 89 clients with myocardial infarction and reported a DVT incidence of 27%. The study also confirmed that DVT is more likely in clients over the age of 60 years with cardiac conditions, such as angina pectoris, left ventricular failure and congestive cardiac failure.

Previous DVT

A past history of DVT in itself is a potent and high risk factor. Residual venous thrombus increases the risk for further acute venous thrombosis.

Incidence of DVT is as high as 68% in patients with a past history of venous thrombosis (Kakkar *et al*, 1970). Nicolaides and Irving (1975) reported a frequency of 61% in clients with previous DVT compared to 26% in clients without a prior history. Clients with previous DVT when exposed to stressful situations, such as surgery, have a four times greater risk of developing new DVT (Dalen *et al*, 1986). In their predictive indexes, Rocha *et al* (1988) and Caprini *et al* (1991) found previous DVT to be a powerful discriminating variable.

Cerebrovascular accident (CVA)

Within a few days of a stroke, 40–53% of patients develop DVT (Warlow, 1978). The DVT occurs exclusively in the paralysed leg and this finding is consistent with 42 chronic hemiplegic patients, where the frequency is also 42%. Physiologically, changes in haemostatic parameters occur after stroke. There is a rise in plasma fibrinogen and an increase in the fibrinogen/fibrin formation. An increased platelet count contributes to blood hypercoagulability. Prolonged immobility whether due to lack of power or sensory loss may apply pressure on the calf and initiate venous thrombosis.

Varicose veins

Anatomically, veins have valves, occurring at regular intervals as shown in Figures 2.3 and 2.4. The valves are arranged so that the blood flow is towards the heart (venous return).

Stretching the veins increases their cross-sectional areas but the valves do not increase in size and, therefore do not close completely. As this develops, the pressure in the veins of the leg increases still further owing to failure of the

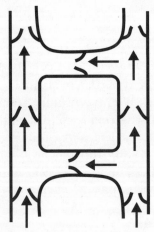 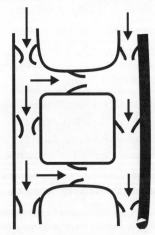

Figure 2-3: Valves in veins   Figure 2-4: Damaged valve and tortuous superficial vein

venous pump, inevitably resulting in venous stasis. Varicosities of the veins cause phlebitis leading to increased risk of DVT. Schaub *et al* (1975) reported a 48% incidence of DVT associated with varicose veins and, in their predictive index, Clayton *et al* (1976) found varicose veins as a clinical characteristic to be a good discriminating factor.

Malignancy

The presence of cancer leads to increased risk of DVT and in post-operative clients, the increase is about 1.5 fold when compared with clients without cancer, regardless of other risk factors (Kakkar *et al*, 1970). It is suggested that the high risk is due to procoagulant substances secreted by the tumour cells, but tumour cells are not usually found in deep veins. Changes in blood viscosity, clotting factors and platelet count are claimed to be responsible but they have not been found to be of pathogenic significance compared to ancillary factors of cancer, such as old age, immobility and major surgery (Kakkar *et al*, 1970; Sue-Ling *et al*, 1986).

Blood groups

Patients with blood group O have been reported to have half the incidence of DVT when compared to those in group A. Jick *et al* (1969) found that group O is under-represented with venous thrombosis compared to that of other blood groups. They also found that group A patients had a higher level than group O patients of antihaemophilic globulin in the plasma. Mourante *et al* (1971) collected and analysed data from 17 studies in connection with blood groups and DVT. They claim that group A has a tendency to thrombose while group O has a tendency to bleed. However, due to the pattern of ABO blood group distribution in the population, the sample in the studies was too small to draw firm statistical conclusions.

Smoking as a risk factor

Cigarette smoking has been blamed for many ills and its implication as a causal factor for DVT is no exception. It is assumed that DVT increases platelet adhesiveness by the release of catecholamines, such as epinephrine caused by nicotine absorption. An alternative explanation is that smoking increases platelet adhesiveness by the release of fatty acids, which may increase the build up of fibrinogen.

The association between cigarette smoking and DVT was first reported by Vessey and Doll (1968). In the study of the relationship between oral contraceptive and DVT, Vessey and Doll (1968) noted that their affected patients were heavier smokers than those in the control subjects. However, the difference between the case and the control group was not statistically significant.

Analysis of cigarette smoking as a clinical variable for DVT demonstrates a negative association (Clayton *et al*, 1976). This report is further supported by Lowe *et al* (1982) who concluded that cigarette smoking is a subjective clinical variable and not a valid predictive index for DVT.

Evidence that cigarette smoking enhances propensity for DVT is without foundation and for this reason is not included as a risk factor in the Autar DVT Scale.

Other associated risk factors

Diabetes has frequently been cited as a risk factor for DVT. It is not certain whether patients with diabetes mellitus have greater risk than non-diabetic subjects. Despite the extensive literature search, there is relatively little substantiated evidence in relation to the association between diabetes and DVT. A frequency of 20% of pulmonary embolism was reported in 349 diabetics aged 30 years or over (Coon, 1976). However, of the 71 patients with PE, 52 had associated heart disease and 12 had other risk factors for DVT. Diabetes predominantly affects the arterial side, especially the microvessels as in retinopathy and nephropathy.

Gender has also been mentioned. However, in hospital men and women were equally affected (Coon, 1976).

The evidence from the above associated risk factors is inconclusive and for this reason, they have not been considered in the development of the Autar DVT Scale.

Summary

- The review of the risk factors in the epidemiology of DVT has provided an awareness of the nature and magnitude of the problem
- Such data should be seriously considered in hospitalised patients
- The risk factors are of practical value in predicting which patients are most likely to develop DVT
- The data can also be used to classify patients into different risk categories
- Surgery, trauma, high risk diseases, increasing age, obesity, immobility, puerperium and pregnancy, oral contraceptives, blood groups and other associated factors have been discussed in terms of their potential for DVT
- These risk factors have been examined to point out the commonality of Virchow's postulates, and to justify their inclusion in developing the Autar DVT Scale
- The study of the risk factors has also highlighted the theoretical perspectives, underpinning the assessment of patients at risk of DVT.

References

British National Formulary (BNF) (1994) *British National Formulary*. No 27. A joint publication of the BMA and the Royal Pharmaceutical Society of Great Britain, London: 301–8

Borrow M, Goldson H (1981) Post-operative venous thrombosis: evaluation of five methods of treatment. *Am J Surg* **141**: 245–51

Brach B, Moser K, Cedar L (1977) Venous thrombosis in acute spinal paralysis. *J Trauma* **17**: 289–93

Caprini JA, Scurr JH, Hasty JH (1988) Role of compression modalities in a prophylactic program for deep vein thrombosis. *Sem Thrombosis Hemostasis* (suppl 14): 77–87

Clayton JK, Anderson JA, McNicol GP (1976) Pre-operative prediction of post-operative deep vein thrombosis. *Br Med J* **2**: 910–2

Coon WW (1976) Epidemiology of venous thromboembolism. *Ann Surg* **186(2)**: 149–64

Crandon AJ, Peel KR, Anderson JA, Thompson V, McNicol GP (1980) Post-operative deep vein thrombosis: identifying high risk patients. *Br Med J* **7**: 343–4

Dalen J, Paraskos JA, Ochene IS, Alpert JS, Hirsh J (1986) Venous thromboembolism: scope of the problem. *Chest* **89(5)**: 370s–73s

DHSS (1982) *Report on Confidential Enquiries into Maternal Deaths in England and Wales 1976–1978*. DHSS 26. HMSO, London

DoH (1994) *Report on Confidential Enquiries into Maternal Deaths in the United Kingdom, 1988-1990*. DoH. HMSO, London

Edwards FC, Truelove SC (1964) The curse and prognosis of ulcerative colitis. *Gut* **5**: 1–15

European Consensus Statement (1991) *Prevention of Venous Thromboembolism*. Med-Orion Publishing, London

Flanc C, Kakkar VV, Clarke MD (1969) Post-operative deep vein thrombosis: effect of intensive prophylaxis. *Lancet* **1**: 477

Freeark RJ, Boswich J, Fardin R (1967) Post traumatic venous thrombosis. *Arch Surg* **95**: 567–75

Goucke CR (1989) Prophylaxis against venous thromboembolism. *Aesth Intens Care* **17(4)**: 458–65

Grace R (1993) Thromboprophylaxis: a review. *Br J Hosp Med* **49**: 720–6

Jick H, Slone D, Westerholm B, Inman WHW, Vessey MP (1969) Venous thromboembolic disease and ABO blood type. *Lancet* 1: 539

Jones DRB, MacIntyre IMC (1975) Venous thromboembolism in infancy and childhood. *Arch Dis Child* 50: 153

Kakkar VV, Howe C, Nicolaides AN, Renney JTG, Clarke MB (1970) Deep vein thrombosis of the legs. Is there a high risk group? *Am J Surg* 120: 527–30

Kierkegaard A, Lars N, Olson CG, Castenfor J, Persson G, Persson S (1987) Incidence of DVT in bedridden non-surgical patients. *Acta Med Scand* 222: 409–14

Lassen MR, Borris LC (1991) Mobilisation after hip surgery and efficacy of thromboprophylaxis. *Lancet* 337: 618

Lowe GD, McArdle BM, Carter DC *et al* (1982) Prediction and selective prophylaxis of venous thrombosis in elective gastro-intestinal surgery. *Lancet*1: 409–12

Madden JL, Hume M eds (1976) *Venous Thromboembolism: Prevention and Treatment*. Appleton-Century-Crofts, New York

Maurer BJ, Wray R, Shillingford JP (1971) Frequency of deep vein thrombosis after myocardial infarction. *Lancet* 2: 1385–7

Miller RC, Lies JE, Caretta RF *et al* (1976) Prevention of lower extremity venous thrombosis by early mobilisation. *Ann Inter Med* 84: 700

Moser KM (1989) Pulmonary thromboembolism: your challenge is prevention. *J Resp Dis* 10(10): 83–91

Mourante AE, Kopec AC, Kazimiera DS (1971) Blood groups and blood clotting. *Lancet* 1: 223

Murray TS, Lorimer AR, Cox F, Lawrie TDV (1970) Leg vein thrombosis following myocardial infarction. *Lancet* 11: 792

Myllynen P, Kammonen M, Rokhanen P (1985) Deep venous thrombosis and pulmonary embolism in patients with acute spinal cord injury: a comparison with patients immobilised due to spinal fractures. *J Trauma* 25: 541–7

Nicolaides AN, Irving D (1975) Clinical Factors and the Risk of Deep Venous Thrombosis. In: Nicolaides AN, ed. *Thromboembolism Aetiology. Advances in Prevention and Management*. MTP Press, Lancaster: 193–204

Nylander G, Semb H (1972) Veins of the lower limb after tibial fractures. *Surg Gyn/Ob* **134**: 974–6

Office of Population Consuses and Surveys (OPCS) (1990) *Mortality Statistics Cause: England and Wales*. A Publication of the Government Statistical Services, DH2, No 17. HMSO, London

Parker-Williams J, Vickers R (1991) Major orthopaedic surgery on the leg and thromboembolism. *Br Med J* **303**: 531–2

Porter JB, Hunter JR, Jick H, Stergachis A (1985) Oral contraceptives and non-fatal vascular disease. *Ob Gyn* **66**: 1–4

Rocha E, Alfaro MJ, Paramo JA, Canadell JM (1988) Pre-operative identification of patients at high risk of deep vein thrombosis despite prophylaxis in total hip replacement. *Thromb Haemost* **59**: 93–5

Rossi EC, Green D, Rosen JS (1980) Sequential changes in factor VIII and platelets in patients with spinal cord injury. *Br J Haematol* **45**: 143–51

Sartwell PE, Masi AT, Arthes FG (1969) Thromboembolism and oral contraceptives: an epidemiological case control study. *Am J Epidemiol* **90**: 365

Sartwell PE, Stolley PD (1982) Oral contraceptives and vascular disease. *Epidemiolog Rev* **4**: 95–109

Schaub N, Duckert F, Fridrich R, Gruber UF, Hay F (1975) Post-operative venous thrombosis. *Langenbeck Arch Chir* **340**: 23

Sevitt S, Gallagher NG (1961) Venous thrombosis and pulmonary embolism: a clinicopathological study in injured and burned patients. *Brit J Surg* **48**: 475–89

Sevitt S, Gallagher NG (1969) Prevention of venous thrombosis and pulmonary embolism in injured patients. *Lancet* **2**: 981–9

Shackford SR, Moser KM (1988) Deep vein thrombosis and pulmonary embolism in trauma patients. *J Intens Care Med* **2**: 87–98

Sharnoff JG, Rosenberg M (1964) Effects of age and immobilisation on the incidence of post-operative thromboembolism. *Lancet* **1**: 845

Silver JR, Morris WR, Ostfinkskowski JS (1980) Associated injuries in patients with spinal injury. *Injury* **12**: 219–24

Simmons AV, Sheppeard MA, Cox AF (1973) Deep venous thrombosis after MI. *Br Heart J* **35**: 623–5

Stamatakis JD, Sagr S, Naird D (1977) Femoral vein thrombosis and total hip replacement. *Br Med J* **2**: 223–5

Sue-Ling HM, McMahon MJ, Johnson D, Philips PR, Davis JA (1986) Pre-operative identification of patients at risk of deep vein thrombosis after elective major abdominal surgery. *Lancet* **1**: 1173–6

Vessey MP, Doll R (1968) Investigation of the relation between use of oral contraceptives and thromboembolic disease. *Br Med J* **2**: 199–205

Vessey MP, Doll R (1969) Investigation of the relation between use of oral contraceptives and thromboembolic disease. A further report. *Br Med J* **3**: 651–7

Vessey MP, Doll R (1970) Post-operative thromboembolism and the use of oral contraceptives. *Br Med J* **3**: 123–6

Warlow C (1978) Venous thromboembolism after stroke. *Am Heart J* **96**(3): 283–5

Wheeler HB (1988) Venous thromboembolism following trauma. *J Intens Care Med* **3**: 65–6

Willen J, Bergquist D, Hallbrook T (1982) Venous insufficiency as a late complication of tibial fracture. *Acta Orthop Scand* **53**: 149–53

Wyshock E, Caldwell M, Crowley JP (1988) Deep venous thrombosis, inflammatory bowel disease and protein S deficiency. *Am J Clin Pathol* **90**: 633–5

Chapter 3

Risk assessment scales

Risk assessment scales are developed to measure an individual's risk status. The recognised risk factors are translated into some quantifiable data which identify the nature and degree of risk. Risk assessment facilitates the application of early and timely intervention which can minimise potential complication or at the very best, prevent its occurrence completely.

An ideal risk assessment tool is one that claims high sensitivity and specificity. When applied to DVT, sensitivity is defined as the percentage of patients who develop and were predicted to develop DVT and specificity is the percentage of patients who do not develop and were predicted not to develop DVT. However, in practice sensitivity and specificity are inversely related: one is achieved at the expense of the other. Despite this limitation of an inverse relationship between sensitivity and specificity, risk assessment tools remain popular, have practical applications and enable a systematic approach to risk assessment. A caution for the use of risk assessment tools is that they are no substitute for clinical decision-making. Nevertheless, when used as an adjunct to clinical judgement, risk assessment tools enhance consistency and predictive accuracy.

Patients' DVT risk assessment status does not usually remain static and fluctuates within a continuum ranging from no risk to high risk (Figure 3.1).

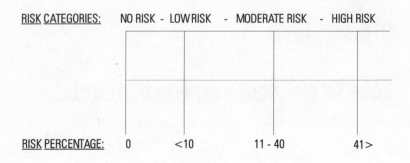

Figure 3-1: DVT risk continuum

DVT risk assessment: the Autar DVT Scale

The Autar DVT Scale as illustrated in Figure 3.2 was developed to:

- Provide a comprehensive nursing assessment tool
- Calculate the degree of risk in an individual, in the context of multifactorial aetiology
- Promote consistency in the professional assessment of practice
- Enable application of preventative measures, commensurate with the category of risk
- Provide quantifiable data for auditing purposes and quality assurance
- Allow the targeting of limited resources
- Create a body of nursing knowledge, embedded in nursing practice.

Autar DVT Risk Assessment Scale

Name
Unit No
Ward

AGE SPECIFIC GROUP

Age group	Score
10-30	0
31-40	1
41-50	2
51-60	3
61+	4

BUILD

Body Mass Index (BMI)
wt(kg) / Ht(m)^2

Build	BMI	Score
Underweight	16-19	0
Average	20-25	1
Overweight	26-30	2
Obese	31-40	3
Very obese	41+	4

MOBILITY

Risks	Score
Ambulant	0
Limited (uses aids self)	1
Very limited (requires help)	2
Chair bound	3
Complete bed rest	4

SPECIAL RISK CATEGORY

Risks	Score
Contraceptive pill (20-35 years)	1
(35+ years)	2
Pregnancy/Puerperium	3

SCORE <6	No risk
SCORE 7-10	Low risk (<10%)
SCORE 11-14	Moderate risk (11-40%)
SCORE >15	High risk (>41%)

SCORING

Identify appropriate items, add and record the scores below

Assessor	Date	Score

TRAUMA RISK FACTORS

Score only preoperatively and score only one item in this box

Risks	Score
Head	1
Chest	1
Head and Chest	2
Spinal	2
Pelvic	3
Lower limb	4

SURGICAL INTERVENTIONS

Minor surgery <30 mins	1
Major Surgery	2
Emergency major surgery	3
Pelvic	3
Thoracic	3
Abdominal	4
Orthopaedic (below waist)	4
Spinal	4

HIGH RISK DISEASES

Risks	Score
Ulcerative colitis	1
Anaemia: Sickle cell	2
Polycythaemia	2
Haemolytic	3
Chronic heart disease	3
Myocardial infarction	4
Malignancy	5
Varicose veins	6
Previous DVT or CVA	7

Figure 3-2: Autar DVT Risk Assessment Scale

The Scale is composed of seven distinct categories of risk factors culled from an extensive literature review of the pathogenesis of deep vein thrombosis. The seven categories are: age specific group, build/body mass index (BMI), mobility, special risk category, trauma risk category, surgical intervention and high risk disease category. The DVT Scale is based on Virchow's triad in the genesis of deep vein thrombosis, which are:

● changes in blood flow due to venous return
● changes in blood composition due to hypercoagulability
● changes in blood vessel wall due to intimal damage.

The guiding principle of the scale is that the risk factors are additive. Each of the risk factors in a category has a unique weighting in terms of its estimated potential for causing DVT. Major or high risk factors have a strong causal consequence, while minor risk factors acting singly are of little or no significance. The risk factors in each category are assigned a relative rating score. Factors carrying little or no risk have a score of 0–1, incrementing to 2 and 3 for low to moderate risk, respectively. A score of 4 or more denotes a high risk factor. A summation of the cumulative effect of all the risk factors provides a discriminatory and prognostic index to DVT. One high risk factor may be present in the low risk clients, rising to 2–4 factors in the moderate category and more than 4 high risk factors in the high risk group (Caprini *et al*, 1988).

How to use the Autar Scale

To calculate a risk category, simply add the scores from each of the appropriate category as applicable to the client. The overall score provides an equation or formula for classifying patients into risk category. The scoring system identifies clients into one of the risk categories outlined in Table 3.1.

Table 3.1: Risk categories

Score range	Risk category
<6	No risk
7–10	Low risk
11–14	Moderate risk
15>	High risk

Most values and tests are not sharply categorised in absolute values but exist on a range of continuous spectrum (Topf, 1986). The scoring range should not therefore replace professional judgement but is another tool to enable nurses to demonstrate consistency and objectivity in the assessment of practice. Further, to demonstrate the practical application of the Autar Scale, four case studies are illustrated in Chapter 4. The incidence of DVT associated with each of the risk categories is illustrated in Table 3.2.

Table 3.2: Incidence of DVT in the risk categories

Incidence (%)	Risk category
<10	Low risk
10–40	Moderate risk
41>	High risk

Source of data: Caprini *et al*, 1988

Risk categories of the Autar Scale

In Chapter 2, the focus of the discussion was on providing a sound understanding of the epidemiology and pathophysiology of deep vein thrombosis. In this section, the intention is to draw on the relevant reviewed theoretical framework to further highlight the rationale underpinning the selection of the seven risk categories of the Autar Scale.

Age specific group

There is a linear relationship between advancing age and the incidence of DVT (Kakkar *et al*, 1970; Nicolaides and Irving, 1975; OPCS, 1990; Wyshock *et al*, 1988). Clayton *et al* (1976) found age to be a powerful discriminatory and reliable predictive factor. Patients over 60 years of age have a high incidence of DVT — 45% (Kakkar *et al*, 1970) — compared with 23% for the 45–59 year-old age group. In children and young adults, DVT is relatively rare with incidence rising after 30 years of age (Coon, 1976). The 10–30 year-old age group carry a score of 0, rising to 4 for those aged 60 years and over.

Mobility

There is a striking relationship between immobility and DVT (Sevitt and Gallagher, 1969; Warlow, 1978; Kierkegaard *et al*, 1987). Immobility causes impairment of venous pump and predisposes to DVT. Early post-operative mobilisation programmes minimise the risk of DVT (Kierkegaard *et al*, 1987). The ambulant patients who are judged not to be at risk have a zero score but for the high risk bedridden patient, the score is 4.

Build/body mass index (BMI)

In this category, patients are broadly classified into one of the five builds according to their body mass index: underweight, average (normal), overweight, obese and very obese. The BMI offers a simple and objective assessment of patients' build derived from the formula: weight (kg) / height (m)^2. Underweight build lies between a BMI of 16–19. The acceptable (normal) BMI range is 20–25. Obesity is taken to start at a BMI of 30 and at 40 for grossly obese patients. A major advantage of a BMI is that the standards are applicable to both male and female patients. A body weight to body mass index (BMI) conversion chart is outlined in Table 3.3. Diminished venous return and some impairment in the fibrinolytic system are reported in overweight and obese patients (Kakkar *et al*, 1970; Poller, 1993).

Table 3.3: Body weight to body mass index (BMI) conversion chart

Height without shoes m	Approx ft in	Significantly underweight (80% of lower end of Acceptable)	Acceptable	Obese	Grossly obese
		Weight (kg) without clothes			
1.45	4.9	34	42–53	63	84
1.48	4.10	35	44–55	66	88
1.50	4.11	36	45–56	68	90
1.52	5.0	37	46–58	69	92
1.54	5.1	38	47–59	71	95
1.56	5.1	39	49–61	73	97
1.58	5.2	40	50–62	75	100
1.60	5.3	41	51–64	77	102
1.62	5.4	42	52–66	79	105
1.64	5.5	43	54–67	81	108
1.66	5.5	44	55–69	83	110
1.68	5.6	45	56–71	85	113
1.70	5.7	46	58–72	87	116
1.72	5.8	47	59–74	89	118
1.74	5.9	48	61–76	91	121

Height without shoes m	Approx ft in	Weight (kg) without clothes			
		Significantly underweight (80% of lower end of Acceptable)	Acceptable	Obese	Grossly obese
1.76	5.9	50	62–77.5	93	124
1.78	5.10	51	63–79	95	127
1.8	5.11	52	65–81	97	130
1.82	6.0	53	66–83	99	132
1.84	6.0	54	68–85	102	136
1.86	6.1	55	69–86	104	138
1.88	6.2	57	71–88	106	141
1.9	6.3	58	72–90	108	144
1.92	6.4	59	74–92	111	147
BMI		<16	20–25	>30	>40

Special risk category

This category applies only to patients who are on contraceptive therapy and in pregnancy and puerperium. Among women taking oral contraceptives, Vessey and Doll (1970) reported a 2.5 greater incidence of DVT in those aged 35–44 than those in the 20–34 age group. For this reason, women in the 20–34 age group are assigned a score of 1 and a score of 2 is assigned to the 35–44 age group.

Cardiovascular changes occur during puerperium. Although the oestrogen levels are considerably reduced during puerperium, they remain higher than normal. The plasma is concentrated and therefore coagulability is increased.

Trauma risk category

Although all patients with trauma carry a risk of DVT (Coon, 1976), those with injury to lower limbs and spinal injury bear the highest risk. The trauma risk category is integrated with the surgical intervention category on the Autar Scale and therefore applies to patients in both surgical and trauma/orthopaedic specialities. However, it must be noted that scoring the trauma risk category only applies to patients pre-operatively or those receiving only conservative treatment for their injuries. The Trauma Risk Category ceases to apply after patients have received surgical intervention for the injury. In brief, either a trauma risk factor or a surgical intervention can be scored at any time. Concurrent scoring inflates the overall score and overpredicts risk.

Surgical intervention

There is a positive correlation between the duration and type of surgery and the increasing incidence of DVT (Borrow and Goldson, 1981). Some surgical procedures are riskier than others in terms of their potential for causing DVT. Orthopaedic surgery (below waist) carries the highest risk with an incidence range of 45–85%, compared to 26% for thoracic and 14–33% for abdominal surgery (Madden and Hume, 1976). Commensurate with incidence risk, thoracic and abdominal surgery have an equal weighting score of 3 each. Orthopaedic procedures carry a rating of 4.

High risk diseases

This category includes inflammatory bowel disease and blood dyscrasias, such as polycythaemia, sickle cell anaemia and haemolytic anaemia. They are associated with increased blood viscosity.

The high risk cardiovascular diseases are chronic heart failure, myocardial infarction, cerebrovascular vascular accident, varicose veins and previous DVT. In this high risk disease category, the score ranges from 1 for ulcerative colitis, rising to 7 for those with previous CVA and DVT. Patients who have had a previous DVT and are now requiring admission are more likely to receive active treatment for their current health problem rather than for their previous DVT. By the very nature of their admission and previous DVT, the aggregate score places such patients into the moderate to high risk category, depending on the number of risk factors present. Table 3.4 illustrates the incidence of DVT associated with some of the high risk diseases and table 3.5 highlights the thrombogenic mechanism of the high risk factors in DVT.

Table 3.4: Incidence of DVT associated with high risk diseases

High risk disease	Incidence (%)	Source of data
Ulcerative colitis	1.3–6.4	Edwards and Truelove, 1964
Polycythaemia	Unclassified	Perkins, 1964
Sickle cell anaemia	Unclassified	Edington and Gillies, 1969
Haemolytic anaemia	Unclassified	Pirofsky, 1969
Chronic heart disease	10–20	Coon, 1976
Myocardial infarction	20–40	Maurer *et al*, 1971
Malignancy	40	Kakkar *et al*, 1970
Cerebrovascular accident	46–53	Warlow, 1978
Varicose veins	56	Kakkar *et al*, 1970

High risk disease	Incidence (%)	Source of data
Previous DVT	68	Kakkar *et al*, 1970 Nicolaides and Irving, 1975

Table 3.5: Thrombogenic mechanism of high risk factors in DVT

High risk factors	Vessel damage	Blood↑ coagulability	Stasis	Fibrinolysis↓
Surgery	+	+	+	+
Leg trauma	+	+	+	
Increasing age			+	
Immobilisation			+	
CVA			+	
Obesity			+	+
Pregnancy/ Puerperium			+	+
Malignancy	+	+		
Oral contraceptive			+	+
Varicose veins			+	
Previous DVT			+	+
Myocardial infarction		+	+	
Heart failure			+	
Polycythaemia			+	
Haemolytic anaemia			+	

High risk factors	Vessel damage	Blood↑ coagulability	Stasis	Fibrinolysis↓
Sickle cell anaemia			+	
Inflammatory bowel disease	+	+		

Summary

- The Autar DVT Scale was developed as a nursing assessment tool for predicting clients at risk of deep vein thrombosis

- Based on Virchow's triad in the pathogenesis of DVT and culled from an extensive literature review and well-founded research findings, the Autar DVT Scale can claim high content validity

- The Scale is composed of seven well-recognised categories of risk factors, namely: increasing age, mobility, build/body mass index, special risk category, trauma, surgical intervention and high risk diseases

- The scoring system identifies the patients with one of the four risk categories: no risk, low risk, moderate risk and high risk. The higher the score, the greater is the risk category.

References

Borrow M, Goldson H (1981) Post-operative venous thrombosis: evaluation of five methods of treatment. *Am J Surg* **141**: 245–51

Caprini JA, Scurr JH, Hasty JH (1988) Role of Compression Modalities in a Prophylactic Program for Deep vein Thrombosis. *Seminar in Thrombosis and Hemostasis* **14**: 77–87

Clayton JK, Anderson JA, McNicol GP (1976) Pre-operative prediction of post-operative deep vein thrombosis. *Bristol Med J* **2**: 910–12

Coon WW (1976) Epidemiology of venous thromboembolism. *Ann Surg* **186(2)**: 149–64

Edington GM, Gillies HM (1969) *Pathology in the Tropics.* Edward Arnold, London: 388

Edwards FC, Truelove SC (1964) The course and prognosis of ulcerative colitis III. *Complications Gut* **5**: 1–15

Kakkar VV, Howe CT, Nicolaides AN, Renney JTG, Clarke MB (1970) Deep vein thrombosis of the leg. Is there a high risk group? *Am J Surg* **120**: 527–30

Kierkegaard A, Norgren L, Olsson CG, Castenfors J, Persson G, Persson S (1987) Incidence of DVT in bedridden non-surgical patients. *Acta Medica Scand* **222**: 409–14

Madden JL, Hume M eds (1976) *Venous Thromboembolism: Prevention and Treatment.* Appleton Century-Crofts, New York

Maurer BJ, Wray R, Shillingford JP (1971) Frequency of deep vein thrombosis after myocardial infarction. *Lancet* **2**: 1385–7

Nicolaides AN, Irving D (1975) Clinical Factors and the Risk of Deep Venous Thrombosis. In: Nicolaides AN ed, *Thromboembolism Aetiology. Advances in Prevention and Management.* MTP, Lancaster: 193–204

Office Population of Censuses and Surveys (OPCS) (1990) *Mortality Statistics Cause: England and Wales.* A Publication of the Government Statistical Services, DH2, No 17. HMSO, London

Perkins J (1964) Polycythaemia vera: clinical studies on a series of 127 patients without radiation therapy. *Q J Med* **33**: 499

Pirofsky B (1969) *Autoimmunisation and the Autoimmune Haemolytic Anaemias.* Williams and Wilkins, Baltimore: 166

Poller L ed (1993) *Recent Advances in Blood Coagulation*, 6. Churchill Livingstone, Edinburgh

Sevitt S, Gallagher NG (1969) Prevention of venous thrombosis and pulmonary embolism in injured patients. *Lancet* **2**: 981–9

Topf M (1986) Three estimates of interrater reliability for nominal data. *Nurs Res* **35(4)**: 253–5

Vessey MP, Doll R (1970) Postoperative thromboembolism and the use of oral contraceptives. *Br Med J* **(3)**: 123–6

Warlow C (1978) Venous thromboembolism after stroke. *Am Heart J* **96(3)**: 283–5

Wyshock E, Caldwell M, Crowley JP (1988) Deep venous thrombosis, inflammatory bowel disease and protein S deficiency. *Am J Clin Pathol* **90(5)**: 633–5

Chapter 4

DVT risk calculation: a practical approach

This chapter examines four clinical profiles and insights into deep vein thrombosis. This approach enables readers to make a practical application of the Autar DVT Scale to the risk calculation of the four clients.

Allow 20–25 minutes to complete the following self-assessment. To check the assessment, turn to pages 63–71.

Autar DVT Risk Assessment Scale

Name	M Bond
Unit No	
Ward	Trauma unit

AGE SPECIFIC GROUP

Age group	Score
10-30	0
31-40	1
41-50	2
51-60	3
61+	4

BUILD

Body Mass Index (BMI)
wt(kg) / Ht(m)^2

Build	BMI	Score
Underweight	16-19	0
Average	20-25	1
Overweight	26-30	2
Obese	31-40	3
Very obese	41+	4

MOBILITY

Risks	Score
Ambulant	0
Limited (uses aids self)	1
Very limited (requires help)	2
Chair bound	3
Complete bed rest	4

SPECIAL RISK CATEGORY

Risks	Score
Contraceptive pill (20-35 years)	1
(35+ years)	2
Pregnancy/Puerperium	3

SCORE <6	No risk
SCORE 7-10	Low risk (<10%)
SCORE 11-14	Moderate risk (11-40%)
SCORE >15	High risk (>41%)

SCORING

Identify appropriate items, add and record the scores below

Assessor	Date	Score

TRAUMA RISK FACTORS

Score only preoperatively and score only one item in this box

Risk	Score
Head	1
Chest	1
Head and chest	2
Spinal	2
Pelvic	3
Lower limb	4

SURGICAL INTERVENTIONS

	Score
Minor surgery <30 mins	1
Major surgery	2
Emergency major surgery	3
Pelvic	3
Thoracic	3
Abdominal	3
Orthopaedic (below waist)	4
Spinal	4

HIGH RISK DISEASES

Risk	Score
Ulcerative colitis	1
Anaemia: Sickle cell	2
Polycythaemia	2
Haemolytic	2
Chronic heart disease	3
Myocardial infarction	4
Malignancy	5
Varicose veins	6
Previous DVT or CVA	7

Self-assessment exercise

Trying out the Autar DVT Scale

Case study one

Mavis Bond, a 71-year-old spinster of average build, has been admitted to the trauma ward of the Trust Hospital. Miss Bond suffers from left ventricular failure which limits her mobility due to breathlessness on exertion. She was negotiating the stairs at home when she lost her footing and, as a result of the fall, sustained a painful and injured left hip. X-rays of the hip confirmed a left fracture neck of the femur with residual osteoporotic change.

To treat her injury, Miss Bond has undergone a total hip replacement. After the arthroplasty, she is maintained on complete bedrest for a week, with her legs positioned in abduction to prevent dislocation of the prosthesis.

Autar DVT Risk Assessment Scale

Name Howard Carruthers
Unit No
Ward Surgical Unit

AGE SPECIFIC GROUP

Age group	Score
10-30	0
31-40	1
41-50	2
51-60	3
61+	4

BUILD — Body Mass Index (BMI) wt(kg) / Ht(m)²

Build	BMI	Score
Underweight	16-19	0
Average	20-25	1
Overweight	26-30	2
Obese	31-40	3
Very obese	41+	4

MOBILITY

Risks	Score
Ambulant	0
Limited (uses aids self)	1
Very limited (requires help)	2
Chair bound	3
Complete bed rest	4

SPECIAL RISK CATEGORY

Risks	Score
Contraceptive pill (20-35 years)	1
(35+ years)	2
Pregnancy/Puerperium	3

SCORE <6	No risk
SCORE 7-10	Low risk (<10%)
SCORE 11-14	Moderate risk (11-40%)
SCORE >15	High risk (>41%)

SCORING

Identify appropriate items, add and record the scores below

Assessor	Date	Score

TRAUMA RISK FACTORS

*Score only preoperatively and score only **one** item in this box*

Risk	Score
Head	1
Chest	1
Head and Chest	2
Spinal	2
Pelvic	3
Lower limb	4

SURGICAL INTERVENTIONS

	Score
Minor surgery <30 mins	1
Major surgery	2
Emergency major surgery	3
Pelvic	3
Thoracic	3
Abdominal	3
Orthopaedic (below waist)	4
Spinal	4

HIGH RISK DISEASES

Risk	Score
Ulcerative colitis	1
Anaemia: Sickle cell	2
Polycythaemia	2
Haemolytic	2
Chronic heart disease	3
Myocardial infarction	4
Malignancy	5
Varicose veins	6
Previous DVT or CVA	7

Case study two

Howard Carruthers is a 55-year-old hotel porter, of overweight build for height and weight (BMI 27). He enjoys good general health and has no record of past medical history, other than a right inguinal hernia which might have been due to occupational hazard, such as lifting heavy loads. He has undergone successful elective repair of the hernia. Following an overnight recovery, Mr Carruthers commences gentle mobilisation and is discharged home.

Autar DVT Risk Assessment Scale

Name: Henry Brown
Unit No:
Ward: **Medical Unit**

AGE SPECIFIC GROUP

Age group	Score
10-30	0
31-40	1
41-50	2
51-60	3
61+	4

BUILD

Body Mass Index (BMI) wt(kg) / Ht(m)^2

Build	BMI	Score
Underweight	16-19	0
Average	20-25	1
Overweight	26-30	2
Obese	31-40	3
Very obese	41+	4

MOBILITY

Risks	Score
Ambulant	0
Limited (uses aids self)	1
Very limited (requires help)	2
Chair bound	3
Complete bed rest	4

SPECIAL RISK CATEGORY

Risks	Score
Contraceptive pill (20-35 years)	1
(35+ years)	2
Pregnancy/Puerperium	3

SCORE <6	No risk
SCORE 7-10	Low risk (<10%)
SCORE 11-14	Moderate risk (11-40%)
SCORE >15	High risk (>41%)

SCORING

Identify appropriate items, add and record the scores below

Assessor	Date	Score

TRAUMA RISK FACTORS

Score only preoperatively and score only use them in this box

Risk	Score
Head	1
Chest	1
Head and Chest	2
Spinal	2
Pelvic	3
Lower limb	4

SURGICAL INTERVENTIONS

	Score
Minor surgery <30 mins	1
Major surgery	2
Emergency major surgery	3
Pelvic	3
Thoracic	3
Abdominal	3
Orthopaedic (below waist)	4
Spinal	4

HIGH RISK DISEASES

Risk	Score
Ulcerative colitis	1
Anaemia: Sickle cell	2
Polycythaemia	2
Haemolytic	2
Chronic heart disease	3
Myocardial infarction	4
Malignancy	5
Varicose veins	6
Previous DVT or CVA	7

60

Case study three

Henry Brown is a 45-year-old postmaster. He is slightly overweight for build: he is 5ft 6 ins tall and weighs around 13 stone. Mr Brown has bilateral varicose veins for which he receives no active treatment other than advice from his GP to keep his legs elevated when at rest.

Mr Brown has had to consult his GP following a sleepless night caused by a painful and swollen left calf. On examination, a positive Homan's sign is elicited: pain in the calf on forceful dorsiflexion. A provisional diagnosis of DVT is made. As a clinical diagnosis of DVT is notoriously flawed (Barnes, 1982), Mr Brown is admitted to the medical ward for objective investigations to confirm the suspected DVT.

Autar DVT Risk Assessment Scale

Name **Michael Dutton**

Unit No

Ward **Surgical Unit**

AGE SPECIFIC GROUP

Age group	Score
10-30	0
31-40	1
41-50	2
51-60	3
61+	4

BUILD
Body Mass Index (BMI)
wt(kg) / Ht(m)²

Build	BMI	Score
Underweight	16-19	0
Average	20-25	1
Overweight	26-30	2
Obese	31-40	3
Very obese	41+	4

MOBILITY

Risks	Score
Ambulant (uses aids self)	0
Limited (requires help)	1
Very limited (requires help)	2
Chair bound	3
Complete bed rest	4

SPECIAL RISK CATEGORY

Risks	Score
Contraceptive pill (20-35 years)	1
(35+ years)	2
Pregnancy/Puerperium	3

SCORE <6	No risk
SCORE 7-10	Low risk (<10%)
SCORE 11-14	Moderate risk (11-40%)
SCORE >15	High risk (>41%)

SCORING
Identify appropriate items, add and record the scores below

Assessor	Date	Score

TRAUMA RISK FACTORS
Score only preoperatively and score only **one** item in this box

Risk	Score
Head	1
Chest	1
Head and Chest	2
Spinal	2
Pelvic	3
Lower limb	4

SURGICAL INTERVENTIONS

	Score
Minor surgery <30 mins	1
Major surgery	2
Emergency major surgery	3
Pelvic	3
Thoracic	3
Abdominal	3
Orthopaedic (below waist)	4
Spinal	4

HIGH RISK DISEASES

Risk	Score
Ulcerative colitis	1
Anaemia: Sickle cell	2
Polycythaemia	2
Haemolytic	2
Chronic heart disease	3
Myocardial infarction	4
Malignancy	5
Varicose veins	6
Previous DVT or CVA	7

Case study four

Michael Dutton is an 18-year-old undergraduate of average build. He has had a recurrent, dull ache and pain in the right iliac fossa for a 'grumbling appendix'. He is now admitted for elective surgery. Following a keyhole appendicetomy completed in less than 30 minutes, Michael makes a good and uneventful recovery. Later, on the operative day, he starts taking fluids and light diet and commences mobilisation under nursing supervision. In the absence of any problem, Michael is discharged home the next day.

Let us review the four clients in the scenarios to check your assessment in relation to their potential risk for developing DVT. The cumulative index of assessment can then be used to identify to which of the four risk categories of the Autar DVT Scale each client should be allocated:

- No risk
- Low risk
- Moderate risk
- High risk.

Recommended preventive interventions for those clients in the low, moderate and high risk categories can be found in Table 4.2, page 80.

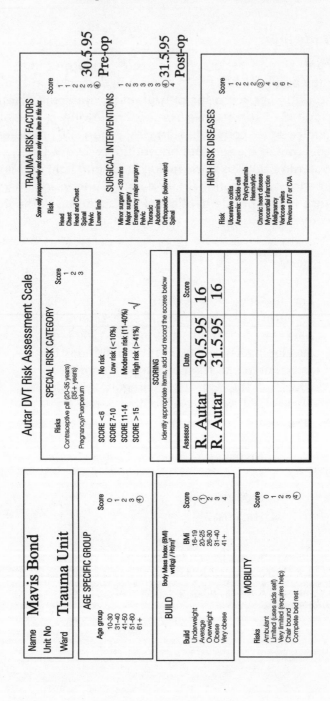

Case study one

Mavis Bond: high risk category

Increasing age is a high risk factor for DVT and Miss Bond, who is in her seventies, fits this category. Although she is of average (normal) build, she has had major, below waist, orthopaedic surgery. Total hip replacement has been associated with a high mortality rate of 17.7% for pulmonary embolism (Sheppeard *et al*, 1981). Of those patients who died from pulmonary embolism, post-mortem evidence confirmed that DVT was the initiator. Miss Bond is on complete bedrest and has an overall score of 16 on the DVT scale. This places her into the high risk category and she has a 40–80% risk of developing DVT and a 1.5% chance of a fatal pulmonary embolism.

Name **Howard Carruthers**

Unit No

Ward **Surgical Unit**

Autar DVT Risk Assessment Scale

AGE SPECIFIC GROUP

Age group	Score
10-30	0
31-40	1
41-50	2
51-60	③
61+	4

BUILD — Body Mass Index (BMI) wt(kg)/Ht(m)^2

Build	BMI	Score
Underweight	16-19	0
Average	20-25	1
Overweight	26-30	②
Obese	31-40	3
Very obese	41+	4

MOBILITY

Risks	Score
Ambulant	0
Limited (uses aids self)	①
Very limited (requires help)	2
Chair bound	3
Complete bed rest	4

SPECIAL RISK CATEGORY

Risks	Score
Contraceptive pill (20-35 years)	1
(35+ years)	2
Pregnancy/Puerperium	3

SCORE <6   No risk
SCORE 7-10   Low risk (<10%)
SCORE 11-14   Moderate risk (11-40%)
SCORE >15   High risk (>41%)

SCORING

Identify appropriate items, add and record the scores below

Assessor	Date	Score
R.Autar	31.5.95	7

TRAUMA RISK FACTORS

Score only preoperatively and score only one item in this box

Risk	Score
Head	1
Chest	1
Head and Chest	2
Spinal	2
Pelvic	3
Lower limb	4

SURGICAL INTERVENTIONS

	Score
Minor surgery <30 mins	1
Major surgery	②
Emergency major surgery	2
Pelvic	3
Thoracic	3
Abdominal	3
Orthopaedic (below waist)	4
Spinal	4

HIGH RISK DISEASES

Risk	Score
Ulcerative colitis	1
Anaemia: Sickle cell	2
Polycythaemia	2
Haemolytic	2
Chronic heart disease	3
Myocardial infarction	4
Malignancy	5
Varicose veins	6
Previous DVT or CVA	7

Case study two

Mr Howard Carruthers: low risk category

Mr Carruthers has had minor surgery, described as one lasting for less than 30 minutes (Borrow and Goldson, 1981). He is overweight for Body Mass Index (BMI) which is considered to be a risk factor. However, he has already commenced gentle ambulation which minimises DVT risk. On the Autar DVT Scale, Mr Carruthers scores 7 and this places him marginally into the low risk category. He has less than 10% risk of developing DVT and less than 0.01% for PE.

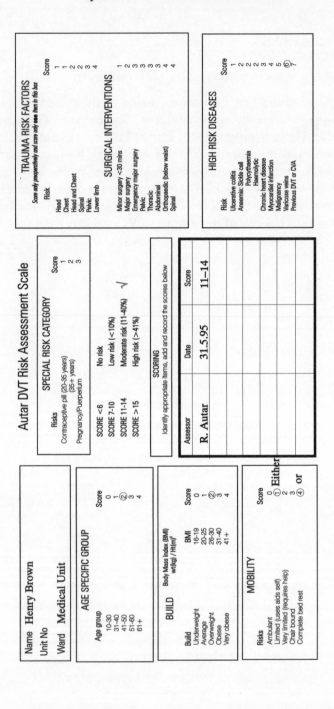

Autar DVT Risk Assessment Scale

Name Henry Brown
Unit No
Ward Medical Unit

AGE SPECIFIC GROUP

Age group	Score
10-30	0
31-40	1
41-50	②
51-60	3
61+	4

BUILD
Body Mass Index (BMI) wt(kg) / Ht(m)²

Build	BMI	Score
Underweight	16-19	0
Average	20-25	1
Overweight	26-30	②
Obese	31-40	3
Very obese	41+	4

MOBILITY

Risks	Score	
Ambulant (uses aids self)	0	
Limited (requires help)	①	Either
Very limited (requires help)	2	
Chair bound	3	
Complete bed rest	④	or

SPECIAL RISK CATEGORY

Risks	Score
Contraceptive pill (20-35 years)	1
(35+ years)	2
Pregnancy/Puerperium	3

SCORE <6	No risk
SCORE 7-10	Low risk (<10%)
SCORE 11-14	Moderate risk (11-40%) ✓
SCORE >15	High risk (>41%)

SCORING
Identify appropriate items, add and record the scores below

Assessor	Date	Score
R. Autar	**31.5.95**	**11-14**

TRAUMA RISK FACTORS
Score only preoperatively and score only one item in this box

Risk	Score
Head	1
Chest	1
Head and Chest	2
Spinal	2
Pelvic	3
Lower limb	4

SURGICAL INTERVENTIONS

	Score
Minor surgery <30 mins	1
Major surgery	2
Emergency major surgery	2
Pelvic	3
Thoracic	3
Abdominal	3
Orthopaedic (below waist)	4
Spinal	4

HIGH RISK DISEASES

Risk	Score
Ulcerative colitis	1
Anaemia: Sickle cell	2
Polycythaemia	2
Haemolytic	2
Chronic heart disease	3
Myocardial infarction	4
Malignancy	5
Varicose veins	⑥
Previous DVT or CVA	7

Case study three

Mr Henry Brown: moderate risk category

Mr Brown has bilateral varicose veins which represents a very high risk factor for DVT. His build is overweight and he has either limited mobility due to the very painful left calf or is immobile due to therapeutic bedrest to prevent dislodgement of the suspected clot. The summation of the cumulative effect of the risk factors for Mr Brown yields a score range of 11–14, subject to his varying level of mobility status. This places him into the moderate risk category. Clients in this category have a 10–40% potential for developing DVT and 0.1– 0.7% for developing fatal pulmonary embolism.

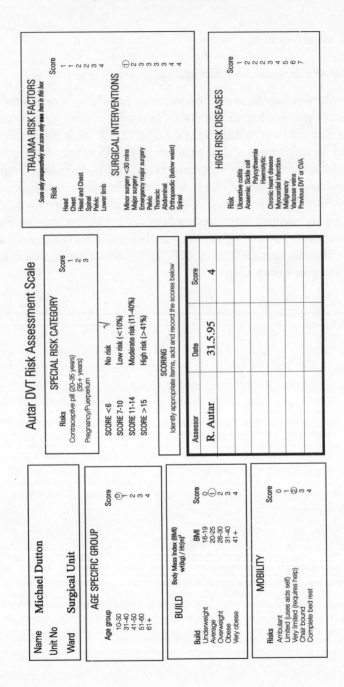

Autar DVT Risk Assessment Scale

Name Michael Dutton
Unit No
Ward Surgical Unit

AGE SPECIFIC GROUP

Age group	Score
10-30	①
31-40	1
41-50	2
51-60	3
61+	4

BUILD
Body Mass Index (BMI)
wt(kg) / Ht(m)²

Build	BMI	Score
Underweight	16-19	0
Average	20-25	①
Overweight	26-30	2
Obese	31-40	3
Very obese	41+	4

MOBILITY

Risks	Score
Ambulant	0
Limited (uses aids self)	1
Very limited (requires help)	②
Chair bound	3
Complete bed rest	4

SPECIAL RISK CATEGORY

Risks	Score
Contraceptive pill (20-35 years)	1
(35+ years)	2
Pregnancy/Puerperium	3

	Score
No risk	✓
SCORE <6	Low risk (<10%)
SCORE 7-10	Moderate risk (11-40%)
SCORE 11-14	High risk (>41%)
SCORE >15	

SCORING
Identify appropriate items, add and record the scores below

Assessor	Date	Score
R. Autar	31.5.95	4

TRAUMA RISK FACTORS
Score only preoperatively and score only one item in this box

Risk	Score
Head	1
Chest	1
Head and Chest	2
Spinal	2
Pelvic	3
Lower limb	4

SURGICAL INTERVENTIONS

	Score
Minor surgery <30 mins	①
Major surgery	2
Emergency major surgery	3
Pelvic	3
Thoracic	3
Abdominal	3
Orthopaedic (below waist)	4
Spinal	4

HIGH RISK DISEASES

Risk	Score
Ulcerative colitis	1
Anaemia: Sickle cell	2
Polycythaemia	2
Haemolytic	2
Chronic heart disease	3
Myocardial infarction	4
Malignancy	5
Varicose veins	6
Previous DVT or CVA	7

Case study four

Michael Dutton: no risk category

There is a positive correlation between the incidence of DVT and increasing age. Only one case of DVT is reported for the 15–19 age group (OPCS, 1990). Michael Dutton has had minor elective surgery, carrying 15% risk compared to 44% for major surgery (Flanc *et al*, 1969; Kakkar *et al*, 1970). It is well-recognised that early ambulation prevents post-operative DVT (Kierkegaard *et al*, 1987). Michael has commenced mobilisation on the operative day. Impaired fibrinolysis is reported in overweight and obese clients compared with their average build counterparts (Kakkar *et al*, 1970; Poller, 1993).

On the Autar DVT Scale, Michael Dutton has an aggregate score of 4 and this places him in the no risk category.

Prevention of deep vein thrombosis: the way forward

Deep vein thrombosis is usually preventable and all patients at risk need to be protected against it. The most cost effective approach to address the problem of DVT is through an aggressive programme of prophylaxis based on identification of patients at risk. Prophylactic management addresses the three factors in Virchow's triad: stasis, vessel trauma and coagulation. The assessment of clients into risk categories as demonstrated by the application of the Autar DVT Scale, facilitates the choice of the most effective prophylaxis as recommended by the European Consensus Statement (1991). A brief review of the prophylactic methods against DVT serves as a reminder that prevention is everyone's business. Thromboprophylaxis can be conveniently divided into physical and pharmacological methods.

Physical methods

Exercise

Stasis in the deep leg veins causes a decrease in mean flow and the pulsativity of the venous flow trace. Exercise is therefore the best and safest method of increasing venous return to the heart. The skeletal muscles' contraction during exercise, particularly the calf, helps to squeeze the leg veins and move blood upwards. During quiet standing, venous pressure at the ankle is 85–90 mmHg. Rhythmic contraction of the leg muscles on exercise lowers the venous pressure to 30 mmHg and so prevents venous stasis (Kaisary, 1982). Both active and passive exercises prevent stasis by promoting venous valve function and muscle action pump (Cotton and Roberts, 1977).

Ambulation and leg elevation

It has long been recognised that early ambulation prevents stasis and thrombi formation (Warlow, 1978; Kierkegaard,1987; Lassen and Borris, 1991). Leg elevation aids gravitational venous return. Ten degrees elevation effects a 30% increase in blood flow velocity (Wolfe and Sabiston, 1980). A recent study by Ashby *et al* (1995) confirms that leg elevation of around six degrees in the supine position aids blood flow and is a simple yet very effective prophylaxis against thromboprophylaxis.

Deep breathing exercise

Deep breathing exercise reduces venous stasis. Alveolar pressure or intrapulmonary pressure is 101kPa or 760 mmHg as in atmospheric pressure at sea level. During inspiration, intrathoracic or intrapleural pressure is 0.5kPa or 4 mmHg

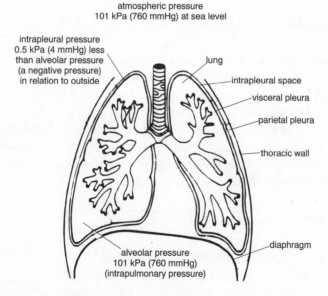

atmospheric pressure
101 kPa (760 mmHg) at sea level

intrapleural pressure
0.5 kPa (4 mmHg) less
than alveolar pressure
(a negative pressure)
in relation to outside

lung

intrapleural space

visceral pleura

parietal pleura

thoracic wall

alveolar pressure
101 kPa (760 mmHg)
(intrapulmonary pressure)

diaphragm

Figure 4-1: Intrathoracic and alveolar pressure

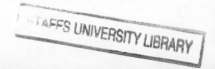

less than alveolar pressure and is called negative pressure. This negative pressure acts as a respiratory suction pump. On inspiration, rising abdominal pressure squeezes the veins and the fall in thoracic and atrial pressure sucks blood back to the heart. Figure 4.1 illustrates the pressure difference between intrathoracic and alveolar pressure.

Graduated compression stockings (GCS)

Graduated compression stockings provide a safe and effective method of prophylaxis against DVT (Alan *et al*, 1983). They apply varying degrees of external compression and work by putting regressive pressure on the vein walls, causing the valvular cusps to come into contact with each other. As a result, the valves become more competent and increase blood flow velocity. Through the application of graduated compression stockings, it is possible to reduce the incidence of DVT in patients undergoing major surgery from 49% to 23% (Holford, 1976).

Intermittent pneumatic compression (IPC)

This pneumatic compression device consists of an air-pump, connecting tubes and extremity sleeves. By the mechanical inflation and deflation of the sleeves, this device promotes blood flow and venous return in the deep veins. By reducing venous stasis it enhances blood clearance from the leg veins and valves sinuses (Scurr *et al*, 1988). IPC also reduces the risk of microtears in the venous endothelium that occur as a result of vascular distension.

Pharmacological methods

The main focus of pharmacological prophylaxis is the use of anticoagulants and antiplatelets. A review of the blood clotting mechanism provides an understanding into the thromboprophylaxis of Heparin, Warfarin and Aspirin.

The blood clotting cascade

Factors promoting coagulation are know as procoagulants
and others inhibiting the process are called anticoagulants.
Following an injury or platelets breakdown, the enzyme
tissue thromboplastin is released. Thromboplastin is a
proteolytic enzyme and it activates prothrombin, converting
it into thrombin. This conversion of prothrombin, a plasma
protein, into thrombin will only occur in the presence of
calcium ions.

Thrombin is a protein enzyme and it acts on fibrinogen,
another plasma protein, converting it into fibrin monomer
and eventually fibrin threads. Fibrin threads form the
reticulum of the clot. The blood clot is a meshwork of fibrin

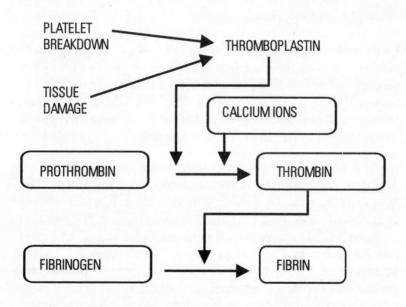

**Figure 4-2: FLOW CHART ONE: The   Normal Blood Clotting
Cascade**

threads, running in all directions, entrapping blood cells, platelets and plasma. The clot initially formed is soft but after a short while, it contracts down and exudates serum, a straw coloured fluid. Figure 4.2 is a schematic representation of the blood clotting cascade.

Antithrombotic drugs

Heparin: is the most widely used anticoagulant. It is now referred to as standard or unfractionated Heparin (UH) to distinguish it from the low molecular weight Heparins (LMWH) which have a longer duration of action. On its own, Heparin has very little anticoagulant effect. However, in the presence of plasma antithrombin III, Heparins inhibit thrombin and so prevent the conversion of fibrinogen to fibrin (Figure 4.3, page 77). Heparins also neutralise activated clotting factor x and therefore prevent conversion of prothrombin to thrombin.

Oral anticoagulant — Warfarin: oral anticoagulants inhibit the synthesis of Vitamin K-dependent coagulation factors. Vitamin K is required to make prothrombin or factors VII, IX and X in the liver. Warfarin, which is the most widely used oral anticoagulant, prevents the manufacture of prothrombin in the liver (Figure 4.3, page 77).

Antiplatelets — Aspirin: the antiplatelet action of Aspirin has long been recognised. Aspirin blocks the synthesis of platelet prostaglandin and inhibits platelets aggregation (Figure 4.3). This prevents clotting. Borrow and Goldson (1981) screened 78 patients receiving 600 mg of Aspirin daily for thromboprophylaxis and reported a DVT incidence of 17.9% (11 patients). Currently, a pulmonary embolism prevention clinical trial (PEP, 1993) is underway to evaluate the efficacy of low dose Aspirin in preventing pulmonary embolism in clients with hip fracture.

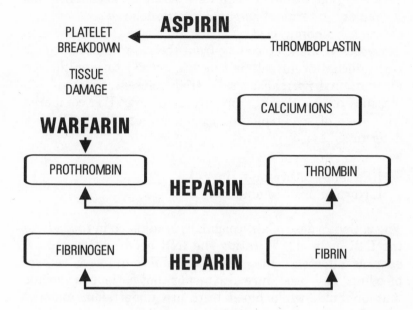

Figure 4-3: Action of antiplatelets and anticoagulants on the Blood Clotting Cascade

Figure 4.3 illustrates the levels where antiplatelets and anticoagulants block the Blood Clotting Cascade. Compare this chart with the Normal Clotting Cascade (Figure 4.2).

● Aspirin prevents platelets aggregation

● Warfarin inhibits the manufacture of prothrombin

● Heparin prevents the conversion of prothrombin to thrombin and so stops fibrin and clot formation.

Cost of anticoagulant therapy

While anticoagulants reduce the body's ability to form clots, they also have low therapeutic index, ie. there are very small differences between the dose required to produce a therapeutic effect and that which produces a toxic effect. This marginal difference can have serious consequences for the patient in terms of personal misery, delayed recovery and the socio-economic cost.

Overdose causes bleeding from the skin, mucous areas and internal organs. It is therfore crucial to monitor the international normalised ratio (INR) closely. The INR is a measure of the patient's prothrombin time (PT) compared with that of a person not taking anticoagulant. INR is determined by:

$$\left[\frac{\text{Patient prothrombin time}}{\text{Normal prothrombin time}} \right]$$

The patient's dose of anticoagulant is adjusted in the light of the INR estimate. Titrating the INR between 2.0 and 3.0 ensures effective anticoagulation and minimises risk of bleeding. This procedure also means that patients are being 'put on hold' while blood tests are undertaken and the adjusted dose of anticoagulant is adminstered. This delay should be avoided and professionals can apply the risk assessment scale and DVT prevention strategies can be implemented.

The safety of patients receiving anticoagulant therapy can be maximised by the health education measures listed in Table 4. 1.

Table 4.1: Advice to patients receiving anticoagulant therapy

* Carry anticoagulant therapy card	
* Attend anticoagulant clinic	
* Take prescribed anticoagulant at the same time daily	
* Remind doctor and dentist of anticoagulant therapy	
* Consult doctors for:	nose bleed/gum bleed/skin bruising
	red or dark urine
	red or dark stool
* Seek advice regarding:	appropriate contraceptive
	starting a pregnancy
* Avoid salicylic preparations (Aspirin) and barbiturates	
* Avoid excessive alcohol	

Self-assessment case studies: recommended preventive interventions

In the earlier self-assessment exercise involving the four case studies, Mr Dutton was deemed not to be at risk and no specific intervention was needed. Varying risk categories were identified for Mr Carruthers, Mr Brown and Miss Bond: low, moderate and high risk respectively. There is a consensus that clients in a particular risk category should receive a recommended prophylaxis for DVT (Caprini *et al*, 1988; European Consensus Statement, 1991; Grace, 1993). Table 4.2 outlines the recommended interventions for the three clients at risk of deep vein thrombosis.

Table 4.2: Strategies in thromboprophylaxis

Risk category	Recommended prophylaxis
Low: Mr Carruthers	Early ambulation Graduated compression stocking (GCS)
Moderate: Mr Brown	Graduated compression stocking + Low dose Heparin or Intermittent pneumatic compression
High: Miss Bond	Graduated compression stocking + Adjusted dose of Heparin Intermittent pneumatic compression

Sources: Caprini *et al*, 1988; European Consensus Statement, 1991; Grace, 1993

Summary

The focus of this chapter has been to demonstrate familiarity with the practical applications of the Autar DVT Scale.

- Four clinical profiles are illustrated to enable readers to evaluate the DVT Scale for its consistency as a risk calculator
- DVT is usually preventable and venous thromboprophylaxis addresses the three factors in Virchow's triad in the causation of DVT
- Prophylaxis against DVT can be achieved by physical and pharmacological methods
- The physical approach includes exercise, early ambulation, leg elevation, deep breathing exercises, the

application of graduated compression stockings and intermittent pneumatic compression

- Heparin, Warfarin and antiplatelets are the preferred antithrombotic drugs
- Although there is no single universal thromboprophylaxis, there is consensus that patients in a particular risk category should receive a recommended prophylactic protocol (Table 4.2).

References

Alan A, Williams JT, Bolton JP, Le Quesne LP (1983) The use of graduated stockings in the prevention of post-operative deep vein thrombosis. *Br J Surg* **70**: 172–4

Ashby EC, Ashford NS, Campbell MJ (1995) Posture, blood velocity in common femoral vein and prophylaxis of venous thromboembolism. *Lancet* **345**: 8947, 419–21

Barnes RW (1982) Current status of non-invasive tests in the diagnosis of venous disease. *Surgic Clin N Am* **62**(3): 484–500

Borrow M, Goldson H (1981) Post-operative venous thrombosis: evaluation of five methods of treatment. *Am J Surg* **141**: 245–51

Caprini JA, Scurr JB, Hasty JB (1988) Role of compression modalities in a prophylactic program for deep vein thrombosis. *Seminars in Thrombosis and Hemostasis* **14(suppl)**: 76–87

Cotton LT, Roberts VC (1977) The prevention of deep venous thrombosis with particular reference to mechanical methods of prevention. *Surgery* **81**: 228–37

European Consensus Statement (1991) *Prevention of Venous Thromboembolism*. Med-Orion Publishing, London

Flanc C, Kakkar VV, Clarke MD (1969) Post-operative deep vein thrombosis: effect of intensive prophylaxis. *Lancet* **1**: 477

Grace R (1993) Thromboprophylaxis: a review. *Br J Hosp Med* **49(10)**: 720-6

Holford C (1976) Graded compression for preventing deep venous thrombosis. *Br Med J* **2**: 968–70

Kakkar VV, Howe CT, Nicolaides AN, Renney JTG, Clarke MB (1970) Deep vein thrombosis of the leg. Is there a high risk group? *Am J Surg* **120**: 527–30

Kaisary A (1982) Let ulcer. Aetiology and pathogenesis of venous leg ulcer. *Nursing* (2nd series) Suppl: 1–7

Kendall Company (1992) *The Guide to Protocol Development for the Prevention of Deep Vein Thrombosis and Pulmonary Embolism*. Kendall Healthcare Products, Europe

Kierkegaard A, Norgren L, Olsson CG, Castenfors J, Persson G, Persson S (1987) Incidence of DVT in bedridden non-surgical patients. *Acta Medica Scand* **22**: 490–14

Lassen MR, Borris LC (1991) Mobilisation after hip surgery and efficacy of thromboprophylaxis. *Lancet* **6**: 337–618

Office Population of censuses and Surveys (OPCS) (1990) *Mortality Statistics causes: England and Wales*. A Publication of the Government Statistical Services, DH2, No 17. HMSO, London

Poller L ed. (1993) *Recent Advances in Blood Coagulation* (6). Churchill Livingstone, Edinburgh

Pulmonary Embolism Prevention (PEP) Trial (1993) *A randomised placebo-controlled trial of the effects of low dose aspirin on mortality and major morbidity in patients with hip fracture*. PEP Trial Office, CTSU, Radcliffe Infirmary, Oxford: 1–18

Scurr JB, Coledridge-Smith PD, Hasty JB (1988) Deep Vein Thrombosis: a continuing problem. *Br Med J* **297**: 28

Sheppeard B, Benson J, Ward DJ, O'Connor (1981) A Clinico-pathological study of fatal pulmonary embolism in a specialist Orthopaedic Hospital. *Arch Orthopaed Trauma Surg* **96**: 283–5

Warlow C (1978) Venous thromboembolism after stroke. *Am Heart J* **96(3)**: 283–5

Wolfe W, Sabiston D (1980) *Pulmonary Embolism*. Saunders, Philadelphia

Chapter 5

Conclusion

Practical application

The DVT Scale effects an approach which is specific to nurses and nursing. It is based on the clinical and demographic data of clients collected routinely by nurses on admission and initial assessment. For thromboprophylaxis to be effective, a comprehensive assessment must be promptly carried out. The Autar DVT Scale facilitates the assessment process within 3–6 minutes (Autar, 1994).

Based on the theory underpinning Virchow's triad of risk factors, the DVT Scale reveals a high content validity and knowledge embedded in practice. This content validity is further supported by the extensive review of literature on risk factors in DVT. Only those factors which are well-founded and clinically proven have been included in the framing of the DVT Scale. It is for this reason that blood group as a risk category was excluded from the scale design. Although A blood group clients are prone to thrombose (Jick *et al*, 1969; Mourante *et al*, 1971), the small analysed data do not allow for firm statistical conclusions to be drawn.

Nurses will have to evaluate for themselves to what extent an assessment tool is applicable to their area of clinical practice. Although the DVT Scale was tried and tested on an orthopaedic unit (Autar, 1994) with favourable results, the design of this assessment tool permits application in diverse clinical areas where DVT is a problem. Age, build and body mass index (BMI) and mobility are intrinsic clinical characteristics common to all clients, regardless of specialities. The other remaining four categories of the DVT Scale cross the boundaries of specialities to address risk assessment of clients in diverse clinical areas. Table 5.1 illustrates the diverse clinical specialities where the incidence of DVT is high and where the DVT Scale can be conveniently applied.

Table 5.1: Diverse clinical specialities

Specialities	Incidence of DVT (%)
Medicine	
Myocardial infarction	10–38
Hemiplegia	33–53
Paraplegia	59–89
Bed-ridden non-surgical patients	13
Surgery	
Major abdominal surgery	3–51
Thoracic surgery	26
Gynaecological surgery	7–45
Prostatectomy	24–51
Orthopaedic surgery	45–74
Neurosurgical patients	29–43

Source of data: Madden and Hume, 1976; Grace, 1993

Consistency/sensitivity/specificity

An ideal risk assessment tool must have consistency, high sensitivity and specificity (Lilienfeld and Lilienfeld, 1980; Mausner and Kramer, 1985).

Consistency

Consistency relates to what extent replication produces similar results. Two measures were applied in two reliability studies, to test the interrater reliability of the Autar DVT Scale: percentage agreement (T%) and Pearson moment correlation coefficient. Percentage agreement was measured by the formula:

$$T\%: \frac{\text{No of agreements}}{\text{No of disagreements}} \times 100$$

The result yielded to a T% of 70–88% for the two reliability studies.

The value of Pearson moment correlation coefficient (r) in both studies achieved a correlation of 0.98 (Autar, 1994).

Sensitivity

Sensitivity is defined as the percentage of those who have the disease (DVT) and in whom it has been predicted (Lilienfeld and Lilienfeld, 1980). Using a cut-off score of 16, the Autar DVT Scale achieved 100% sensitivity and 81% specificity (Autar, 1994).

Specificity

Specificity is defined as the percentage of those who do not have DVT and in whom this has been predicted (Lilienfeld and Lilienfeld, 1980). Although an 81% specificity was obtained, in clinical practice, sensitivity and specificity are inversely related. A high sensitivity (100%) is achieved at the expense of specificity (81%) and alteration in the cut-off score can alter the sensitivity and specificity of an instrument.

Developing the Autar DVT Scale in practice

With any risk assessment tools, including the Autar DVT Scale, nurses must not be complacent but should exercise professional judgement to complement the use of these tools. Before an instrument from the professional market is allowed into general circulation, clinicians must ensure that it has been tested for the theory it purports to support (Cormack and Reynold, 1992). A battery of rigorous testing is necessary. As instruments undergo a process of validation in diverse clinical areas and new information comes to light, they should be modified accordingly. The Norton Pressure Sore Risk Assessment Scale (1962) is a classic example of an instrument that has undergone scrutiny and change. Gosnell (1973) modified it and later Norton (1987) herself adapted it so that the scoring system is reversed: the higher the score, the greater is the risk. The same treatment should apply to the Autar DVT Scale. It is likely that diverse clinical specialities and centres using the Autar DVT Scale, by the nature of their diversity, may find that the threshold score of 16 used in the initial study is not the best discriminator of those 'at risk'. It is therefore recommended that nurses using the Autar DVT Scale should evaluate the best cut-off score to enhance predictive accuracy. After all, it is only accurate risk assessment that will enable the targeting of appropriate resources and effective interventions. Finally, future studies should also focus on differences between clients who develop DVT and those who do not. Additional data can then be analysed to compute those discriminatory variables or risk factors which are most significant.

Summary

- The Autar DVT Scale has a practical application. Its clinical and demographic variables are data routinely gathered on the admission of a client
- For thromboprophylaxis to be effective, a prompt and comprehensive assessment is necessary and the Autar DVT Scale facilitates this process
- The design of the Scale encourages its application in diverse clinical specialities where DVT is a threat
- The Autar DVT Scale has shown reliable consistency, sensitivity and specificity as a predictive index
- Clinicians should evaluate the DVT Scale in terms of the best threshold score to enhance predictive accuracy.

References

Autar R (1994) *Nursing assessment of clients at risk of deep vein thrombosis: The Autar DVT Scale*. Unpublished MSc Dissertation. University of Central England in Birmingham

Cormack DFS, Reynolds W (1992) Criteria for evaluating the clinical and practical utility of models used by nurses. *J Adv Nurs* **17**: 1472–78

Gosnell DJ (1973) An assessment tool to identify pressure sores. *Nurs Res* **22**: 55–9

Grace R (1993) Thromboprophylaxis: a review. *Br J Hosp Med* **49(10)**: 720–6

Jick H, Slone D, Westerholm B (1969) Venous thromboembolic disease and ABO blood type. *Lancet* **1**: 539

Lilienfeld AM, Lilienfeld DE (1980) *Foundation of Epidemiology*, 2 edn. Oxford University Press, Oxford: 150–9

Madden JL, Hume M eds (1976) *Venous Thromboembolism: Prevention and Treatment*. Appleton Century-Crofts, New York

Mausner JS, Kramer S (1985) *Epidemiology. An Introductory Text*. W B Saunders Co, Philadelphia

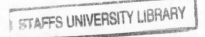

Mourante AE, Kipec AC, Domaniewska-Sobczak K (1971) Blood groups and blood clotting. *Lancet* **1**: 223

Norton D, McLaren R, Exton-Smith AN (1962) *An Investigation of Geriatric Nursing Problems in Hospitals*. National Corporation for the Care of Old People, London

Norton D (1987) Norton revised risk scores. *Nurs Times* **83 (41)**: 6

Glossary

Antihaemophilic globulin:
- A blood clotting factor also known as factor VIII. It is one of the coagulants used for treating haemophilia

Antithrombin III:
- An alpha globulin and one of the most important anticoagulants that removes thrombin from blood

Arthroplasty:
- The surgical remodelling of a diseased joint

Body mass index (BMI):
- An individual weight and height which allows the determination of ideal weight. The BMI is used to define the nutritional status as well as to determine whether an individual is underweight, obese or very obese. It is derived from the formula: weight (kg)/height (m)^2

Blood dyscrasia:
- An abnormal condition of the blood or bone marrow, such as anaemia, leukaemia or Rh incompatibility

Epidemiology:
- The study of the determinants and distribution of disease in the human population

Euglobulin lysis time (ELT):

- This test measures the ability of the patient's plasma to lyse or dissolve precipitated euglobulin. Dissolution of fibrin by a patient's plasma confirms the presence of free circulating plasmin

Fibrinolysis:

- A system which is responsible for the dissolution of fibrin clot

125/Fibrinogen scanning:

- Leg scanning for DVT involves the incorporation of fibrinogen labelled with radio-active iodine into the thrombus. The labelled fibrinogen is detected by measuring the increase in overlying surface activity with an isotope detector

Homan's sign:

- Pain is experienced in the calf by the patient on forceful dorsiflexion. It is clinically diagnostic of DVT

Haemolytic anaemia:

- Excessive destruction of red blood cells, resulting in anaemia. The red cells are unduly fragile and therefore more easily destroyed

Pathogenesis:

- The origin and development of a disease

Prothrombin time:

- Prothrombin is one of the clotting factors (factor II). Prothrombin time is the time required for a coagulation to take place. Normal prothrombin time is approximately 12 seconds

Puerperium:
- It is the period of time after childbirth, up to about six weeks, when the size of the womb decreases to normal

Polycythaemia:
- This rare disease is characterised by overactivity of the haemopoetic tissue, resulting in an increase in the red blood count

Sickle cell anaemia:
- This is a severe form of anaemia due to abnormality of haemoglobin in red blood cells, leading to sickle-shaped cells in the blood stream

Thromboembolism:
- A blood clot formed at one point in the circulation becomes detached and lodges at another point

Thrombocytosis:
- An increase in the number of platelets in the blood. It is likely to cause increased tendency to clot formation

Venography:
- This is an invasive technique involving the injection of a contrast medium directly into the foot. An X-ray is then taken to follow the course of this medium in its passage up the leg

Abbreviations

BMI:

- Body mass index

CVA

- Cerebrovascular accident

DVT

- Deep vein thrombosis

GCS:

- Graduated compression stocking

IBD:

- Inflammatory bowel disease

ICD:

- International Classification of Disease

INR:

- International normalised ratio

IPC:

- Intermittent pneumatic compression

LDH:

- Low dose Heparin

LMWH:

- Low molecular weight Heparin

NIH:

- National Institute of Health

OPCS:

- Office of Population Censuses and Surveys

ORIF:

- Open reduction internal fixation

PE:

- Pulmonary embolism

PEP:

- Pulmonary embolism prevention

PT:

- Prothrombin time

UH:

- Unfractionated Heparin

Deep vein thrombosis: the silent killer

Index

Fibrinogen 75–77
Fibrinolysis 16–17, 26,
47, 51–52, 90
Fibrins 16–17, 75–77
Fibrinogen scanning 26, 90

Glossary 89–91
Glycocalyx 15–16
Graduated Compression
Stockings 10, 74, 80
Gynaecological surgery 21,
84

Haemolytic anaemia
(see anaemia)
Head injury 22, 43
Heart disease 30–31, 43,
50–52
Hemiplegia (see also CVA)
31–32
Heparin 10, 76–77
Hernia 59
Homan's sign 6, 90
Hypercoagulability 8, 18, 28

Immobility 19, 26–28, 51
Inflammatory bowel
disease 30
Injuries; head 22, 43
chest 22, 43
pelvic 22, 43
spinal 23, 43
Intermittent pneumatic
compression 10, 74, 80
International Classification
of Disease 24–25
Intrathoracic pressure 73

Malignancy 33

Perforators 2
Phagocytes 5
Pharmacological methods
74–80
Phlebosclerosis 25
Plasma protein C 16
Plasmin 17
Plasminogen 17
Pneumatic compression
device (see intermittent
pneumatic compression)
Polycythaemia 30
Postphlebitis syndrome 4
Pregnancy/puerperium
2 9–30
Prithrombin 75–78
Prothrombin time 78
Pulmonary embolism 4

Recanalisation 5
Risk   assessment
scales
Risk factors; 19
blood groups 33
contraceptives 28–29
diabetes 34
high risk diseases 30–33
immobility 26–28
increasing age 24–25
obesity 25–26
pregnancy/puerperium
29–30